DR MANDELL'S LIFETIME ARTHRITIS RELIEF SYSTEM

Dr Marshall Mandell is medical director of the New England Foundation for Allergic and Environmental Diseases and head of the Alan Mandell Center for Bioecologic Disease. He is the author of the bestselling *Five Day Allergy Relief System,* published by Arrow, and co-author of *The Mandell's It's Not Your Fault You're Fat Diet,* and lives in Connecticut. He is a fellow of the American College of Allergists, of the International Academy for Preventive Medicine, of the Society for Clinical Ecology and of the Academy of Orthomolecular Psychiatry. He was formerly Assistant Professor of Allergy at New York Medical College and is now Adjunct Professor of Allergy and Nutrition at the University of Bridgeport. He was recently awarded the prestigious Forman gold medal for his original research into arthritis and allergies of the nervous system.

DR MARSHALL MANDELL

Dr Mandell's Lifetime Arthritis Relief System

ARROW BOOKS

Arrow Books Limited
17-21 Conway Street, London W1P 6JD

An imprint of the Hutchinson Publishing Group

London Melbourne Sydney Auckland
Johannesburg and agencies
throughout the world

First published in Great Britain 1984

© Marshall Mandell M.D. 1983

Set and printed in Great Britain by
The Guernsey Press Co. Ltd.
Guernsey, C.I.

ISBN 0 09 934810 1

To the memory of—

Albert and Beatrice Mandell who took me into their home, gave me their name, their love, and worked long and hard to give me the medical education that has made this labor of love possible.

My beloved son, Alan Michael, who created so much beauty in his all too brief twenty years.

Herbert Rinkel, M.D., and Michael Zeller, M.D., who "opened the door" to new medical horizons for all of us.

To the millions of arthritis victims whose months and years of pain, despair, and crippling could have been lessened, eliminated, or prevented.

To the millions who, now, today, can be spared the tragedy of unnecessary suffering and deformity by the application of well-established bioecologic methods of diagnosis and treatment.

To all my fellow physicians—caring and compassionate healers—whose Hippocratic Oath, personal integrity, and professional obligations to their patients require that, in their unending search for truth, they look beyond the present unsatisfactory drug-oriented state of mainstream medical practices. And, with open minds, I hope that they will independently make their own objective observations and form conclusions regardless of existing prejudices, misinformation, and pressure from the medical establishment.

To my mentor and wise friend, Theron G. Randolph, M.D., the father of Clinical Ecology, whose monumental contributions to human welfare have changed the course of medical progress. His brilliant concepts and steadfast, uncompromising dedication to the very best in the practice of rational medicine have been an inspiration to all who are privileged to know him.

Contents

Author's Note   9
Foreword I, by Theron G. Randolph, M.D.   11
Foreword II, by William Kaufman, Ph.D., M.D.   15
Preface by Roger J. Williams, Ph.D.   17
Introduction: The Bioecologic Approach to Arthritis   19

Section I   Arthritis and Allergy

1. "Thank You for Giving Me Back My Health"   25
2. What Is Arthritis?   41
3. Standard Treatments for Arthritis   53
4. What Is "Allergy"?   63
5. How Allergies Cause Arthritis   79

Section II   How to Relieve Allergic Arthritis

Before You Begin . . .   91
6. Finding Clues to Your Allergy-Related Arthritis   95
7. How to Free Your System from Arthritis-Causing Substances   133
8. The Six-Day Rotary Diagnostic Diet   173
9. How to Identify and Control the Environmental Causes of Your Arthritis   185
10. The Lifetime Arthritis-Relief Diet   217
11. Nutrition and Arthritis   237
12. Finding Help—Doctors' Attitudes—Laboratory Tests   249
Epilogue   262
Index   264

Author's Note

My readers are privileged to read the prefatory comments of three distinguished scientists of world reknown who have honored me by sharing their experiences and thoughts on this very common, painful, and often crippling disease. I sincerely thank each of them for his most welcome contribution to this book.

I also wish to express my gratitude to my respected medical friends and colleagues who so kindly supplied me with data from their office and hospital records along with their important observations, clinical impressions, and conclusions based on thousands of patient-years of practice.

I especially want to thank my friends Thurman Bullock, M.D., and Murray Carroll, M.D., of Chadbourn, North Carolina; Harris Hosen, M.D., of Port Arthur, Texas; Kendall Gerdes, M.D., of Denver, Colorado; William Kaufman, Ph.D., M.D., of Stratford, Connecticut; George Kroker, M.D., of LaCrosse, Wisconsin; Joseph J. McGovern, Jr., M.D., of Oakland, California; Joseph Morgan, M.D., of Coos Bay, Oregon; Theron G. Randolph, M.D., of Chicago, Illinois; William Rea, M.D., of Dallas, Texas; Phyllis Saifer, M.D., of Berkeley, California; and Jacob Siegel, M.D., of Houston, Texas; for providing me with excellent case histories that give additional, independent clinical confirmation that firmly establishes the allergy-arthritis connection.

Their much appreciated and most generous cooperation has provided me with more case histories than space has permitted me to present. I sincerely thank them for their efforts to help me enlighten arthritis sufferers, those who care about them, and the health professionals who treat them.

A warm and friendly word of thanks to those great patients—mine and those of my colleagues—who gave their time, efforts, and thoughts to help others. Their cooperation in preparing additional information and going that extra mile in checking and rechecking our results has earned them a special place in medical progress and in the thoughts of many, many people they will help but never meet.

To my caring, deeply involved, and hardworking office staff, for all their valued assistance to me and the patients we are privileged to serve, a heartfelt thank-you and well done. Their very special individual contributions to the welfare of others go far beyond the competent discharge of their assigned duties.

This note of acknowledgment would be incomplete without my heartfelt thank-you to three special ladies—my wife, Fran, for her patient understanding; Sara Gilbert, who helped organize the information; and my very much appreciated executive secretary and research coordinator, Joan Jewell, who helped me in so many ways.

Foreword I

Millions of arthritics are being denied optimal medical care by rheumatologists and many other so-called arthritis experts, because of their persistence in applying long-accepted but relatively ineffective medical approaches to this disease. The tragedy and the largely unnecessary pain inherent in this statement are underscored by the fact that the demonstrable roles of common foods in arthritis was clearly stated over three decades ago.[1,2] Since this time these clinical observations have been confirmed repeatedly and extended to include the ability of various environmental chemical exposures to induce and perpetuate arthritis.[3]

A cooperative study of rheumatoid arthritis of the hands was recently carried out by three participating environmental-control hospital units. A total of forty-three patients were studied before and after a preliminary period of fasting and avoidance of probable environmental causes of chronic arthritis.* Both subjective reports and objective measurements of grip strength, joint tenderness as measured by means of a dolorimeter index and joint circumference (arthrocircometer measurements) were checked before and follow-

* Probable environmental causes of chronic arthritis were "avoided" because exposure to particles of airborne allergens and various sources of indoor air pollution were controlled to the greatest degree possible. This control is achieved by the design, construction materials, furnishings, and overall operation of the in-hospital ecology units, including the activities. clothing, cosmetics, and the like of the entire professional and maintenance staffs.—AU.

ing test reexposures. Highly significant findings, including a decline of grip strength, an increase in joint tenderness, and an increase in the swelling of involved finger joints, occurred following the test ingestion of organically grown specific foods and exposure to selected environmental chemicals. The frequency of major, severe, adverse reactions was highest for cereal grains and meats. Approximately one half the patients tested for reactions to the cumulative intake of chemical additives and contaminants of the diet also experienced a recurrence of arthritis and other reactive symptoms, whereas the same foods in their organic form had been tolerated. Selected patients also experienced a measurable recurrence of arthritis to burning natural gas, formaldehyde fumes, phenol, volatized synthetic ethyl alcohol, and certain other environmental chemicals. Details of these clinical observations have been submitted for publication.[4]

Why then have most rheumatologists and other physicians failed to apply this ecologically oriented medical approach? There seems to be no simple answer. But a combination of the following points seems to account for this retarded acceptance and application of clinical ecology to the management of arthritis.

Modern medicine has become progressively *mass-applicable* and less individualized as it depends increasingly on laboratory tests in diagnosis and on drug therapy for suppression of symptoms. Traditionally, medicine has remained *bodily centered* in contrast to environmentally focused. Prodded by desires to cut costs and save time, mass-applicable medicine, characterized by *a*nalytical, *b*odily *c*entered and *d*rug-related programs, has become the rule. Although this *ABCD* approach has been helpful in handling many acute illnesses of short duration, it has been relatively ineffective in many chronic illnesses such as arthritis. Many patients react adversely to drugs used in the treatment of arthritis.

Medicine needs to be more *individualized* and *e*nvironmentally *f*ocused to be maximally effective in the diagnosis and treatment of arthritis. Building on the above *ABCD* program and minimizing the use of drugs, a more effective environmentally oriented program for arthritis is expressed by the acronym *ABC(D)EF* of individualized medical care—the medical approach of clinical ecology.

Clinical ecology may be described as an offshoot of allergy, in the original broad sense of this term, and toxicology. Its development fills a long-neglected medical-environmental void between these areas as they are usually applied. The distinctive features of clinical ecology will become apparent as you read this book.

Whether this relatively new medical field is practiced on an office or hospital basis, it depends on the demonstration of cause-and-effect relationships as patients are challenged with environmental materials. Acute, highly significant reactions may be induced experimentally, which establish the environmental relationships of the patient and this person's illness. For example, if the arthritis in a patient is related to the intake of foods, avoidance of such a food will be helpful. Symptoms reappear when reexposed to such a food or foods.

At least 90 percent of patients with rheumatoid arthritis may be helped significantly by the application of this medical approach, providing the patient follows through with the recommended program in his or her case. Under these circumstances, the type of program recommended in this book should be tried first rather than last or never in the management of arthritis.

Unfortunately, the precise mechanisms as to why the techniques of clinical ecology work are not well understood as yet. The fact remains that management of arthritis based on the identification of offending materials is a workable approach which should be applied far more widely, even though the underlying mechanisms are not understood.

—THERON G. RANDOLPH, M.D.

Notes for Foreword I

1. M. Zeller, "Rheumatoid Arthritis—Food Allergy As a Factor," *Annals of Allergy* (1949) 7:200.

2. H. J. Rinkel, T. G. Randolph, and M. Zeller, *Food Allergy* (Springfield, Ill.: Thomas), 1951.

3. T. G. Randolph, "Ecologically Oriented Rheumatoid Arthritis," in *Clinical Ecology,* ed. L.D. Dickey (Springfield, Ill.: Thomas), 1976, p. 201.

4. R. T. Marshall, et al., "Comprehensive Environmental Control and its Effect on Rheumatoid Arthritis: I. Fasting; II. Food and Chemical Challenges," unpublished.

Foreword II

Dr. Marshall Mandell is a physician, an allergist, a clinical ecologist, a clinical researcher, an author, and an excellent public communicator in his chosen field. He has written this book to show how unsuspected allergies can cause the troublesome symptoms and signs of "allergic arthritis," including joint discomfort, pain, stiffness, swelling, and impaired joint mobility.

Dr. Mandell explains how he uses special techniques to pinpoint the allergy-causing foods and environmental materials that can cause allergic arthritis in a susceptible person. Once these allergens are eliminated from the person's diet and environment, there is recovery from allergic arthritis. Then, as a final test, when Dr. Mandell reexposes such a patient to the offending allergens, the allergic arthritis recurs. This completes the cycle of clinical proof that these specific allergens have caused the individual's allergic joint illness. When these allergens are excluded on a long-term basis, the patient again recovers from allergic arthritis.

The types of patients with allergic arthritis described by Dr. Mandell are not rare. They are seen by general practitioners, internists, pediatricians, and arthritis specialists. The diagnosis of arthritis is easily made but an allergic origin is rarely suspected or explored. As a result, the first treatment the patient receives is usually a heavy daily intake of aspirin or one of the new drugs that acts like aspirin. This helps relieve pain, discomfort, and stiffness but unfortunately may also cause unpleasant side effects. Although drug treatment may add to the patient's comfort, it fails to remove the allergenic cause of the patient's joint problem. In contrast, Dr. Mandell's treatment removes the allergenic cause so that drug treatment is unnecessary.

A patient with severe osteoarthritis or a patient with rheumatoid arthritis may have joint symptoms and signs based on the underlying disease process. However, in both these situations, in susceptible patients, allergens may worsen the overall arthritis by superimposing allergic joint symptoms and signs. And elimination of the specific allergens may confer major relief from joint symptoms not obtainable by drug treatment alone.

In the past, many physicians have properly diagnosed and successfully treated allergic arthritis by eliminating offending allergens from the patient's diet and environment. Dr. Mandell has built on the clinical experiences of such physicians, adding his own important and unique contribution in furthering clinical knowledge about the diagnosis and treatment of allergic arthritis.

Whatever the reason, it is only fair to say that many reputable doctors do not believe that allergic arthritis exists. However, the existence of this condition is not a matter of belief. That allergic arthritis exists is a demonstrable fact.

—WILLIAM KAUFMAN, PH.D., M.D.

Preface

Marshall Mandell, M.D., though he has traditional medical training, has become so interested in arthritic disease in relation to the nutritional process that he challenges his colleagues to do something about it.

This is a most potent challenge and has at least three sets of facts which contribute to its reasonableness. One of these sets of facts is the existence of a large number of nutritional essentials, the interplay of which may enter into the etiology of arthritic disease. The second set has to do with the large number of substances which can act as allergens and can cause serious metabolic disorder. The third set of facts has to do with the ubiquitous presence of biochemical individuality in all members of the human family.

Biochemical individuality in the metabolic realm is so prevalent that it is estimated that there may be thousands of genetic aberrations widespread in the population. Presumably these would yield to metabolic manipulation if we knew how to do it.

Obviously, in the light of the three sets of facts cited above, the nutritional treatment of arthritic disease is not a simple matter. The fact that we do not yet know what the important nutritional factors in arthritis may be is relatively meaningless because we have made so few sophisticated trials in this and other areas. Nutritional science is really in its infancy.

The most promising development, which suggests that the nutritional challenge may be met within a reasonable time, is the extensive experience and investigation of Dr. John Ellis and Professor Karl Folkers and his associates on the carpal tunnel syndrome. This syndrome certainly has something to do with arthritis.

—ROGER J. WILLIAMS, PH.D.
March 31, 1982

Introduction

The Bioecologic Approach to Arthritis

If you are among the over 35 million Americans enduring the pain, physical limitations, and emotional stress brought on by arthritis, it is very likely that this book can help you. You owe it to yourself to read its message. The self-help techniques of diagnosis and treatment described here can offer considerable relief—and perhaps complete elimination—of your pain, swelling, and stiffness.

If you are among the millions more who have a friend or relative suffering from arthritis, this book offers the opportunity to share with them a message of health and hope. For a majority of them there *is* a way to relieve arthritis—one that is simple and free from the potentially dangerous side effects of drugs. There is a biologically sound way to relieve pain and stiffness and to prevent crippling before repeated attacks lead to permanent, irreversible damage.

Even those arthritic individuals who already have painful deformities can often be helped. For many the pain and swelling can be significantly reduced or eliminated by this method, and the progression of deformities can in most cases be completely arrested.

What you read in this book may be questioned and perhaps criticized by some members of the medical establishment. Most of my fellow physicians are only slowly, if at all, coming to recognize the serious disorders of our bodies and minds that are caused by what we eat, drink, breathe, and absorb each day. Rheumatologists—"arthritis specialists"—and the Arthritis Foundation itself acknowledge that they do not know the cause for arthritis and therefore cannot be sure of its prevention or cure. Yet they respond to inquiries from the arthritic patient with information that may involve complex and expensive courses of medication and treatment. These therapies work only for some of the people some of the time. They have, almost without exception, uncomfortable and at times dangerous side effects. And they can be costly not only in terms of money but in terms of the quality of a patient's life.

"Live with it" is too often the only advice offered to arthritis sufferers. "We'll operate in a few years," a rheumatologist may predict; that is, *after* "a few years" of potentially hazardous drug, chemical, and even radiation treatment!

Clinical ecologists, on the other hand, approach the problem of arthritis from a different viewpoint. Clinical ecologists and bioecologists are medical doctors who study and treat the effects of environmental factors—the foods and beverages we ingest, including the chemicals that are added to them or contaminate them; airborne allergens like house dust, animal dander, pollens, and molds; chemical pollutants of indoor and outdoor air; and other stress factors—on our patients' total physical and mental health.

We say: "Until we thoroughly investigate all the various possible causes of arthritis in each person's diet and environment, we cannot identify and properly treat the specific factors responsible in any given case. Therefore, instead of adding a potentially harmful, chemically derived drug to burden the already-present stresses in an arthritic person's body, let's work along with each patient to identify accurately the specific causes of the particular illness by reproducing the symptoms and then eliminating or controlling the substances that are aggravating that person's allergically reactive muscles and joints." Instead of saying, "You must learn to live with it," we want you to change your diet and the way you live—sometimes just a little. Working on this serious health problem together, there is an excellent chance that we can relieve or eliminate your arthritis.

Through the pioneering work of Dr. Michael Zeller and Dr. Theron G. Randolph over three decades ago and the work of their colleagues and students, many thousands of arthritis sufferers have been greatly relieved of or freed from pain, and crippling deformities have been prevented or reduced in severity or cured. Evidence from their research and my own has established that in the vast majority of cases, arthritis is caused by allergic and allergylike reactions to commonly ingested foods and beverages as well as often-encountered natural or synthetic environmental chemicals and/or the natural airborne substances that many people are allergic to.

Eighty to 90 percent of patients whose chronic illness has been investigated using the ecologists' diagnostic approach to arthritis have clearly been shown to be suffering not from an "unexplainable" disease due to "unknown causes" but from a series of frequently occurring adverse reactions to generally unsuspected and overlooked everyday substances.

Comprehensive allergic-ecologic management of the underlying causes of the illness has improved the condition of most sufferers from this painful and potentially crippling disease. By carefully following my self-help lifetime system, you should be able to obtain the welcome relief from arthritis that others have achieved as outpatients in the office practice of ecologically oriented physicians or in environmentally controlled hospital ecology units.

Section I presents actual documented case histories and research findings from my files and those of my fellow ecologists. These case histories will help you understand what arthritis is, what we ecologists mean when we use the term *allergy*—and how the two are connected.

Section II will show you how to identify and control or eliminate the factors that you may be exposed to often—perhaps daily—in your own environment that may be causing your arthritis or that of a loved one. By following the outlined techniques carefully, thoroughly, and with the appropriate precautions, many people afflicted with arthritis will now be able to provide their own relief—quickly, safely, and in many cases, permanently.

Chapter 12 will direct you to sources for further help and information, whether you simply want to know more about arthritis and the new and growing field of clinical ecology and bioecologic medicine or feel the need for finding professional help. Don't worry if you can't do it *all* on your own. You can locate clinical ecologists through their national society, or you can refer to the ecologic medical centers listed in chapter 12, where diagnostic tests and comprehensive, nondrug methods of treatment have proven to be effective for thousands of arthritis sufferers.

Section I

Arthritis and Allergy

1

"Thank You for Giving Me Back My Health"

In October of 1981 a woman from New Hampshire spent a few weeks under my care at the Alan Mandell Center for Bio-Ecologic Diseases in Norwalk, Connecticut. She described herself as "very much in pain day and night due to arthritis in my hands and shoulders. I had not slept through a full night in months. I could not even wash my own hair because my shoulders were so painful."

One month after we had diagnosed her problem as an allergic reaction to certain foods, including refined cane sugar, she says she found herself "a hundred percent free of pain, sleeping through the night, and my energy level has increased tremendously.

"It is pure joy to walk with the living again," she writes. "Thank you for giving me back my health." Her thanks for my efforts and those of my office staff are very gratifying. It is also gratifying that she now knows enough about the causes of her illness to be able to manage her arthritis on her own. She knows that in one sense she is not permanently "cured," but that she can stay in full control of her chronic joint disease by following the individualized, special diet that was prescribed for her after our symptom-duplicating food tests showed us exactly what foods, beverages, and additives caused her allergic arthritis.

An orthopedic surgeon is discovering for himself the enormous value of allergically and ecologically oriented arthritis control. Dr. Robert Samuelson Ford of the Midwest had been practicing orthopedic surgery for about twelve years and leading an active, athletic life when he began to have pain in his hip and shoulders. Over the next few years of unnecessary suffering and emotional stress, the stiffness and discomfort became so severe that he had trouble sleeping and walking. His thigh muscles were so badly affected that he actually had to walk backward very slowly when going down a flight of stairs. Diagnosed as having rheumatoid arthritis, he underwent a series of treatments with aspirin, cortisone, and gold injections. Although he had occasional remissions, his overall condition worsened to the point that he could no longer perform surgery due to his extreme fatigue and the stiffness in his hands. He told me that it was impossible to do hip surgery any longer because he did not have the physical strength to stand in the proper position for the duration of the procedure or to move the patient's thigh on the operating table. He was forced to give up an important part of his practice due to pain and exhaustion.

After ten years of agony he learned almost by accident of the wonderful results being achieved in Dr. Theron G. Randolph's environmentally controlled ecologic unit for allergic diseases in Chicago. When I spoke with Dr. Ford in September, 1981, he had been in Henrotin Hospital under the care of Dr. Randolph's associate, Dr. Richard S. Wilkinson, for eighteen days. All his arthritis medications had been discontinued, and after the first few days of a five-day spring-water fast, he began to be able to move freely without pain. By the end of the fast, he was able to move his hands almost well enough to perform surgery again, if he only had the stamina for it.

He was undergoing a series of carefully selected single-food diet tests that provoked diagnostically invaluable acute attacks of arthritis that duplicated in every respect the symptoms of his chronic illness. (The details of this method of testing will be described in Section II.) He had already learned that one of his major food sensitivities was to corn. A few hours after eating a bowl of cooked cornmeal with corn syrup, he reacted as follows: "I just started hurting . . . like being kicked by a mule . . . it lasted twelve to fifteen hours." Another very severe reaction was to chicken. After eating a portion of this popular food, he "took a nap," which might have been an acute episode of uncontrollable allergic fatigue, and in a while this victim of allergic arthritis woke up crying, the pain was so severe. "I was weeping. And I consider myself tough . . . it was brutal." He told me that potatoes gave him "a lesser reaction, but a quick one" that came on rapidly and cleared within a few hours.

Within a few weeks Dr. Hall had learned he could be free from his arthritis symptoms by eliminating all foods at once while on the spring-water fast. He also had an opportunity to learn painfully that single-food provocative-feeding tests for the foods he was eating on a regular basis had dramatically induced acute flare-ups of his familiar chronic and disabling arthritis. And these flare-ups positively could not be called spontaneous, since they were related to the deliberate ingestion of specific foods.

Although his friends and colleagues in the medical profession had vigorously tried to discourage him from seeking controversial eco-logic diagnosis and treatment from Dr. Randolph and his associates, Dr. Ford learned the truth about his arthritis. His painful allergic muscles and allergic joints that had made him so miserable for so long were inflamed by food tests and relieved by fasts. The reader should keep in mind the fact that Dr. Ford is a specialist in diseases of the musculoskeletal system, and he is now thoroughly convinced of the role of allergy in severe forms of rheumatoid arthritis.

Another doctor formally reported to her colleagues on the staff of a North Carolina hospital her happy experience in finding allergy and arthritis relief through an ecologic investigation which proved that unsuspected and unrecognized allergy was the sole cause of many long-term disorders she had been afflicted with. She had lived for years with a variety of physical ailments that physicians labeled as psychosomatic, with fatigue and depression that psychiatrists had diagnosed as an emotional illness, and with arthritis that had pro-gressed to the point of causing bone damage to her feet. Although she was often in too much pain to walk, she—as had many other highly allergic patients with bodywide allergy—had finally begun to believe that perhaps her multiple-system, multiple-symptom illness really was all in her mind. That's how it was until she came under the care of Dr. F. Murray Carroll and Dr. Thurman Bullock, clinical ecologists at the Southeastern Chronic Disease Center in Chadburn, North Carolina. Under their expert care, she was tested for a variety of food sensitivities and showed an especially strong arthritic reac-tion to cane sugar, a potent and frequent cause of symptoms that some traditional allergists do not recognize as an allergen.

By removing all offending foods and the sugar from her diet, Drs. Carroll and Bullock were able to cure her so-called hypochondria. Although the probably avoidable bone deformities in her feet cannot be altered by diet, she now lives without the severe arthritic pain that had greatly limited her life. She reports, a little embarrassed, that whenever she succumbs to her lifelong fondness for sweets, her aching joints make her pay for it.

These are not miracles. They positively are not what the medical establishment calls spontaneous remissions. They only underscore the validity of the bioecologic approach, which tests for and identifies allergic sensitivities to environmental factors that cause allergic (bioecologic) arthritis and removes the patient from contact with the culprits—allergens and chemical substances we come into contact with daily. This system often provides almost immediate relief from many kinds of allergies, including allergy-based arthritis. Those who experience and witness this relief may consider it a miracle, but it is biologically sound medical practice based on the cause-and-effect method of diagnosis and treatment, as doctors themselves realize when they learn of it firsthand. No intelligent, clear-thinking layman or physician can resist its beautiful logic. Don't cover up the symptoms—find the cause!

It is interesting that Dr. Thurman Bullock himself, now director of the ecology unit at the Columbus County Hospital in North Carolina, was a general practitioner who became involved in ecologic medicine as the result of his wife's successful ecologic treatment for arthritis. She and Dr. Bullock noticed that every time she was hospitalized for tests or treatment for her arthritic condition, it improved, but that it worsened soon after her return home. The young rheumatologist in charge of her case concluded that these remissions away from home were emotional, due to the protective environment of the hospital. However, Dr. Bullock made the connection between the limited diet she consumed by habit at home and the much more varied menus she selected when in the hospital and away from her own kitchen. Her system had become overloaded with foods to which she had become allergically sensitive as a result of her habitual, monotonous diet. As soon as she began to eat a larger number of foods in a planned sequence, her arthritis was relieved. Rotating the ingestion of a diversified group of foods prevented the buildup of an allergic overdose of any single food.

Over the last decade Dr. Bullock and Dr. Carroll have successfully treated numerous cases of allergic arthritis in the rheumatoid, osteo, and other forms, which will be described in the next chapter. Among them:

A fifty-six-year-old bookkeeper with gout, rheumatoid arthritis, and other arthritis-related symptoms who was advised to discontinue all medications (which had done little good for many years) and placed on a diet that avoided eggs, carrots, celery, bananas, and papaya. Result: no more arthritis.

A fifty-four-year-old schoolteacher who was nearly disabled despite heavy doses of Bufferin and cortisone demonstrated allergic sensitivity to ten foods, including eggs, strawberries, and coffee, which were eliminated from her diet. Result: 95 percent relief from pain (with no medication) for four years except for flare-ups when she was deliberately or accidentally exposed to the food allergens.

A thirty-year-old woman with a history of milk allergies during infancy and four years of pain despite arthritis medications was given a diet free from milk and all milk products. Result: no medication, no pain, no complaints—no arthritis.

Sometimes the allergy-arthritis response is sudden, obvious, and dramatic. For instance, one of my patients, a severely arthritic middle-aged woman, experienced relief of her painful symptoms through the elimination of milk from her diet. Under double-blind laboratory conditions, when milk was introduced to her system sublingually, she immediately became extremely tired, weak, and achy. She felt severe pain in most of her joints, especially her hips, which were much too uncomfortable for her to move about.

For a patient of Dr. Harris Hosen, who employs the ecologic technique at St. Mary's Hospital in Beaumont, Texas, one of the major culprits was orange juice. She was a seventy-six-year-old woman with a six-year history of severe arthritis who lost all her pain, stiffness, and disability while fasting on spring water in a controlled environment under Dr. Hosen's care. She experienced almost immediate pain and trembling when she took a drink of orange juice after completing her fast. "It knocked me for a loop," she told me. Her other doctors had said, "You are getting old, and arthritis is an incurable disease. We may have to operate in a few years." She reported, "They never did mention that food might cause it." After a few days of fasting, the arthritic joints of her right shoulder, elbow, and wrist had improved so much that she was able to reach around and touch the back of her neck for the first time in years. She did react to several other foods, but orange juice was the worst offender.

Sometimes the roots of the problem are a little harder to dig out. A patient came to me after years of fruitless drug treatment under the care of rheumatologists. From her history it was clear that she was allergy-prone. A week-long fast at home that almost eliminated all her arthritis symptoms proved that her arthritis was in large part due to food allergy. But it took a lot of testing to discover all her arthritis-causing dietary sensitivities, as they included almost two dozen foods of a wide variety, from bananas through ham and peanut butter to tuna fish.

A sixty-one-year-old patient at the Southeastern Center had a long history of various disorders, including heart trouble, intestinal problems, diabetes, and arthritis, for which he had found no relief through conventional treatments. It took Drs. Carroll and Bullock a great deal of effort to pinpoint the entire spectrum of his food sensitivities, since they were many and wide ranging. But once these sensitivities were identified and removed, all his arthritis and intestinal problems disappeared. Since his food allergies were so numerous, he is being treated with desensitizing injections of food extracts to enable him to eat a number of the foods he is allergic to.

In most cases, allergic arthritis can be controlled by adjustments in the diet or changes in the environment, as case after case from over the years, from around the country and abroad, demonstrates.

For example, a nurse in her mid-thirties developed arthritis in her hands, feet, knees, and shoulders that was so severe she could walk only with the aid of crutches. After a few days of fasting in Dr. Theron G. Randolph's environmentally controlled ecology unit in Chicago, she was free from the swelling, inflammation, and pain in her joints. As, one by one, she was tested with a series of single-food ingestion challenges and then exposed to a variety of household chemicals, it became clear from her reactions which substances had caused her allergic arthritis. By eliminating and avoiding some of those chemical substances that polluted her home environment as much as possible and rotating her diet through an individualized diet consisting of a group of safe foods (by a simple process I will later describe), she was able to resume her career and her life as a wife and mother.

A musician whose arthritis became so severe that it was endangering her career noticed that it often eased when she was on tour but returned when she was in her own home. The cause was found to be the natural gas with which her home was heated and with which she cooked. She had an overall sensitivity to all petroleum-related products, in fact, and when she began cooking and heating with electricity and wearing natural-fiber clothing instead of petroleum-derived polyesters, her arthritic condition improved dramatically and her hands regained the flexibility necessary to play her violin.

Over a period of twelve years a businessman's arthritis grew so disabling that he could walk only with crutches. Drugs were doing nothing to impede the progression of his crippling pain, but a short period in an environmentally controlled hospital brought marked improvement. Tests of foods and chemicals revealed that he was sensitive to milk, beef, and some grains as well as to natural gas. In the years since, by regulating his diet and installing electric heat, he has been able to pursue an active life on and off the job, and enjoys a variety of vigorous sports.

A nine-year-old child with juvenile rheumatoid arthritis who underwent a knee operation after aspirin treatments failed to relieve her condition was finally brought to Dr. Randolph when even surgery had not helped. Her condition cleared up rapidly during a fast, but she suffered severe recurrences of arthritic pain following the reintroduction of a variety of foods that were eaten in a series of single-food test meals. She was also found to be sensitive—chemically susceptible—to the fumes of natural gas. Now, with a carefully regulated, individualized diet and a gas-free home, she lives a completely normal childhood, except for receiving physiotherapy on her knee—a direct result of the fruitless and unnecessary operation. The bioecologic approach is to identify and treat the cause, not to remove tissues surgically that can be healed.*

In mid-July of 1982, as the manuscript of this book was undergoing its final revision, a very sweet fifteen-year-old, Jennifer, was carried in her father's arms from her wheelchair into my consultation room. This intelligent, lovely teenager is the crippled victim of conventionally treated juvenile rheumatoid arthritis. She is unable to walk or bend her elbows, and she uses her handicapped hands with moderate difficulty.

To date, during the initial phase of her ecologic investigation, we have been able to flare up some of her familiar joint pains during provocative testing with allergenic extracts prepared from carrot and brewer's yeast. The symptoms caused by her arthritis-duplicating tests were reversed (relieved or neutralized) by the symptom-relieving technique of Dr. Carleton F. Lee, an early researcher in the field of clinical ecology, which further establishes these foods as very likely factors in her

*These case reports were kindly supplied by Dr. Theron G. Randolph.

disabling illness. I now have positive confirmation of the role of these arthritis-provoking foods in this case because Jennifer has had a Rinkel deliberate single feeding test for each of these foods and both yeast* and carrot have caused predicted—not "spontaneous"—exacerbations of her arthritis.

Testing has also shown that she probably suffers abdominal pain from house dust and milk, headache from auto exhaust, barley, and hormodendrum (a mold), left hip pain from lettuce, generalized itching and fatigue from chlorine, a moderately dazed condition from corn, severe nausea and hiccups from natural gas, moderate pain in the right hip and both knees from carrot, and severe pain in the right hip extending to the right thigh from brewer's yeast. These familiar, long-term symptoms were induced by sublingual provocation tests. Different substances tested brought on different patterns of symptoms.

Comprehensive ecologic management cannot loosen her contractions or dissolve the ankylosis in her joints, but I hope that we can prevent further pain and damage by blocking future exacerbations of her chronic illness. And if it should flare up in the future, we will apply emergency ecologic measures in a hospital-based environmental-control unit. We will do this by directly attacking simultaneously all the demonstrated and probable causes of this miserable and tragic disorder.

One cannot turn the clock back, but it is impossible for me to look at this appealing and uncomplaining young lady and not wonder what she might be like today if someone had advised Jennifer's parents to bring her to Dr. Randolph, or to any ecologist who is fortunate enough to have a forward-looking hospital that permits or encourages the diagnostic and treatment methods of clinical ecology, before this terrible disease left its mark on her.

Case after case from my own files and those of other ecologists demonstrates the connection between allergies—food and environmental sensitivities—and arthritis. Each of these patients suffered the usually prolonged, painful symptoms of arthritis. Most of them had undergone the standard drug therapies, from aspirin and more powerful drugs to gold injections and steroids, to no avail. Yet all of

---

*A yeast-containing vitamin product was immediately discontinued and her hip pain (which interfered with her sleep) was decreased considerably and she was able to sleep through the night for the first time in months. Her parents were very pleased with this welcome benefit from their daughter's allergic-ecologic investigation of her arthritis.

them found rapid relief as soon as their particular offending allergens were pinpointed and removed from their diets and their environments. It is also highly significant that during the course of their treatment for arthritis, other generally recognized symptoms of allergy—for example, runny nose, itching, sneezing, coughing, and rash—also cleared up. Their arthritis was only one of several allergic reactions to the same substance(s) that affected their muscles and joints.

One of the typical frustrating experiences of a bioecologist's professional career occurred when I was working in the allergy clinic of a local hospital. The patient was a woman suffering from allergic bronchial asthma. She said that she would try to keep the next appointment we had made for her, but it might be difficult because she also had appointments to visit an internist at the medical clinic for her "emotional" spastic intestinal problem (colitis), at the urology clinic for her frequent episodes of bladder symptoms that did not seem to be caused by an infection (frequent, urgent, and uncomfortable urination), at the dermatology clinic for her itching skin rash (eczema), and at the neurology clinic for her recurring migraine headaches.

I tried to explain to her that a series of special tests for bodywide allergies in my office might very well identify the causes of *all* those problems, but I could not convince her. I was left exasperated by the clinical repercussions brought about by overspecialization within the medical profession. Each of the doctors in the various clinics, though well trained and competent within his or her own area of expertise, was looking at only one aspect of an illness with many facets. The specialists did not see the whole patient as an individual with closely interrelated, malfunctioning organ systems within one body and were fractioning it instead of seeing it as a whole and responding as a whole.

Modern physicians are not instructed in clinical ecology and do not recognize or suspect the presence of highly individualized, patient-specific, bodywide reactions to various substances in the diet and the environment—reactions that take place often at the same time in different organs. The lack of a bioecologic orientation in the current practice of medicine brings to mind the story of the five blind men who came up with five different interpretations of the structure of an elephant's body, depending on the part they happened to touch, which, in turn, depended on where they happened to be standing at the time.

Dr. Hosen reports the case of a woman who was receiving

successful therapy for allergic headaches and nasal trouble. He learned that for two years she had also been suffering joint pain, which her physician diagnosed as rheumatoid arthritis. Why had she not mentioned this before? She "did not want to bother Dr. Hosen with her troubles," she told him, and she "knew it could not be due to an allergy." Dr. Hosen had her temporarily eliminate the foods that she usually ate and placed her on a diet consisting of foods that she usually did not eat—an individualized, food-elimination diet. Very soon she was completely free of arthritis. She was then given a series of single-food ingestion tests to identify her arthritis-causing foods. When this very easy case of dietary allergic arthritis was fully understood, she was cured by an extremely simple nondrug, nonsurgical measure—removing tomatoes from her diet!

Dr. Hosen's case of "tomato arthritis" should not be misinterpreted as clinical evidence supporting Dr. Childer's conclusion that foods which are members of the nightshade family have a more important role in the causation of arthritis than members of other food families. When Dr. Hosen challenged this patient with a single-food test feeding of potato, a very important nightshade vegetable, no arthritis symptoms were provoked.

This observation clearly shows that there is a very definite, and extremely important, difference in the response of an arthritic joint after the ingestion of two foods in the same botanic family—tomato and potato. Some arthritis-evoking factor (or factors), present in tomato—and absent in potato—is/are absorbed and carried by the circulation to the arthritic joint after being released from the food source during digestion.

The following brief case report involves a member of the gourd family. Dr. Hosen's case of tomato arthritis reminded me of one of my favorite patients, a middle-aged woman whom I affectionately named "Cucumber Annie." Mrs. R. had moderately severe arthritis for a number of years, and in reviewing her diet, I learned that it had been her custom to have a daily cucumber salad for many years. And I certainly was not surprised to learn that she loved to eat cucumbers. By now, you have already guessed "the rest of the story." Her favorite salad vegetable, a member of the melon, squash and pumpkin family of gourds, was responsible for her arthritis. At my suggestion, the cucumber salad was eliminated and the joint problems cleared, but they reappeared when she ate "cukes," pickles or pieces of pickled cucumbers in relish, tartar sauce or Thousand Island salad dressing.

Dr. Jacob Siegel of Houston, Texas, treated an elderly nurse with a long history of allergic respiratory illness who always carried three pairs of shoes to work because "her feet had been most painfully troublesome." She found it only slightly helpful if she changed her shoes several times during a work shift, but she was never really comfortable. Dr. Siegel's testing elicited a positive reaction to chicken and her consumption of this food was then greatly restricted. In his letter to me he noted: "The pain in her feet disappeared; her joy and gratitude were immense."

He described a case of possible arthritis in a 27-year-old man whose hands were swollen and stiff, "each the size of a baseball catcher's mitt." Beef was identified as an offending food and a reduced intake of same "resulted in a complete resolution of his presenting symptoms." There also was "other system involvement," as is so often the case with allergic disorders. There was "complete reversal of extremely severe constipation which had required continuous medication since the age of two. His elimination became normal."

A patient with ankylosing spondylitis that almost completely disabled him was tested for allergies by Dr. Siegel. This patient stated that he feels his back stiffening up "just like the Tin Man in *The Wizard of Oz*" when he ingests some of the foods to which he has been found allergic.

Joseph J. McGovern, Jr., M.D., of Oakland, California, has contributed the case of a 35-year-old woman with "disabling rheumatoid arthritis (RA) involving all joints of the fingers and the wrists of both hands." The illness of several years duration had become severe about three and one-half months previously "and had not responded to medication. In order to determine the cause of the RA, the patient was placed on a six-day fast, followed by a single-food re-feeding schedule. Ninety minutes after the ingestion of corn," there was a significant flare-up of her arthritis that "coincided with the highest recording of immune complexes (90) . . . nine times above normal range (0-10) . . ."

This laboratory information is mentioned here because some reader might wish to inform his internist or rheumatologist that Dr. McGovern* has demonstrated a direct relationship between an extremely important series of laboratory findings and an exacerba-

*Your physician may contact Dr. McGovern at 400 29th Street, Oakland, California 94609.

tion of RA immediately following the ingestion of a major food offender. He wrote that I "can be sure that nobody else in the world has," at the present time, "this kind of data," which combines the fasting-food-testing-provoked arthritis flare-up and the immunologic and biochemical changes that confirm the fact that an important series of reactions occurred as a result of food allergy.

The following situation often occurs: patients who seek treatment for skin, eye, digestive or respiratory conditions that they know or strongly suspect are allergies will, unexpectedly, and to their very pleasant surprise, find that they are also freed from other long-term complaints that often include muscle and joint symptoms (arthritic aches, pains, swelling and stiffness) they had not realized were allergic in origin.

Dr. Siegel writes, "We must be sure that patients with arthritis have all had complete, intensive medical investigation to make sure that the arthritis is not a symptom of any disease. In the great majority of such patients, there also are symptoms in other body systems that the patient will not report because they do not feel that such other symptoms are relevant. One often finds multiple system symptomatology, where all X-ray and laboratory tests are negative.

"Where, in addition to the arthritis, there are also respiratory, gastrointestinal tract symptoms, skin complaints, chronic fatigue, cerebral symptoms, such as headaches, insomnia, postprandial (after eating) somnolence, depression, learning disability, etc., then a common denominator such as allergy must be considered."

Dr. Carleton Lee of St. Joseph, Missouri, one of the leading research-oriented physicians in clinical ecology (now retired), recently informed me that of the more than fifteen thousand patients he has seen during the last twenty years, only 1 percent of them came to him for treatment of their arthritis. Most of those thousands of patients did not even mention joint or muscle symptoms when reporting their various allergic complaints. To his great surprise, Dr. Lee found that *40 percent* of his fifteen thousand patients did have some form of arthritis in addition to their other allergies.

With cause-directed allergy treatment consisting of desensitizing shots, individualized special diets, and comprehensive environmental control, arthritis disappeared along with the hay fever, asthma, itching, red eyes, chronic nasal and sinus disorders, blocked ears, and headaches. In addition, many other unrecognized allergic problems the patients had suffered from for years—without realizing they were allergic manifestations—also responded to ecologic management.

Many patients had lived with their arthritis for so long that they accepted it as "one of those things that just happen to people" and they no longer gave much thought to their aches and stiffness until they suddenly found themselves free of these discomforts. Interestingly, Dr. Lee's own seasonal arthritis was completely relieved by allergic management of his weed-pollen sensitivity.

I have often encountered similar situations, and happy coincidences have occasionally included other members of the patient's family in my own practice. In one coincidence I was testing a ten-year-old child who had asthma and hay fever, and I found her asthma was made worse because of her sensitivity—chemical susceptibility—to natural gas. Fumes from the kitchen stove were the only source of gas in her home. I instructed the family to have the stove removed, and soon after the child's home was free of gas fumes, her mother, who had never been a patient of mine, noticed that her arthritis had completely disappeared. As soon as I learned of this unexpected and most welcome bonus, I asked Mrs. S. to come to my office for a test to detect petrochemical sensitivity. We tested Mrs. S., using Dr. Randolph's special technique for demonstrating chemical allergy that employs petroleum-derived alcohol, and almost immediately brought on a flare-up of her usual arthritis manifestations.

The characteristic clinical course of arthritis, with its "unpredictable" mysterious flare-ups due to "unknown causes" and so-called spontaneous remissions, actually gives us some important clues to its allergic nature because it comes and goes like other exposure-dependent allergies. For instance, an arthritic person for whom aspirin has been providing satisfactory relief may experience a sudden attack of his usual joint and muscle symptoms as autumn approaches. He or she might assume (or be told) that the colder weather might have somehow touched off this episode of arthritis. However, it is not likely that the lower temperature is responsible for many arthritis flare-ups, although there are some people who suffer from thermal food allergy. (This is an allergic condition in which cold weather or chilling lowers the allergic person's allergic resistance to foods they are capable of reacting to.)

The environmental factors I consider if a patient's arthritis symptoms are intensified in autumn include the following:

1. Internal effects caused by absorption of arthritis-producing factors from inhaled airborne pollens released from local weeds and

late-pollinating grasses. It is not widely known that highly reactive grass pollens can cause considerable allergic trouble during the ragweed season. On many occasions I have noted that the local grass-pollen count has been higher than the weed-pollen count during weed-pollen season.

2. At this time of year the atmosphere can be loaded with the enormous quantities of reproductive spores and broken threads of many species of very potent molds. Substances in these molds can also be absorbed internally from the moist surfaces they come in contact with and ultimately reach the allergically sensitive cells in the joints and muscles that are involved in cases of mold-allergy arthritis.

3. The house is now closed to conserve heat; this causes an increase in the concentration of several types of allergenic substances in indoor air, such as house dust, dust mites, pet dander, and molds—in addition to the odors of cooking foods and the chemical fumes of a variety of maintenance materials employed in housekeeping, and the gassing out from synthetic furnishings, cosmetics, and volatile, odorous materials employed while engaging in hobbies.

4. When nonelectric heating systems are turned on, the combustion products of fuel oil, natural gas, kerosene, coal, or wood may pollute the indoor environment. In addition, the blower in a hot-air heating system distributes airborne offenders of many types throughout the house.

Another example of the signs of allergy-based arthritis is that of a man who suffers flare-ups of his familiar pain and stiffness while on the job but not when he is away on vacation. His personal physician or a consulting psychologist or psychiatrist might suspect that there are arthritis-causing stresses at his place of work, and his doctor or the consultant might recommend that he find different employment, with fewer physical and emotional demands. Based on my experience, I would advise a very careful search of the workplace for the presence of inhalant allergens and reactive airborne chemical substances—dust in the heating ducts, janitor's supplies, cosmetics, tobacco smoke, potted plants with moldy soil, odorous furnishings, and fume-generating equipment—to which he is sensitive.

To discover the ecologic causes of your own arthritis, you must join me and my colleagues and become a self-employed ecologic detective. Section II will provide a wealth of clues that will prepare you for this fascinating detective work. For now it will be enough for you to give considerable thought to many aspects of your problem and consider a few important questions.

If you are now under treatment for arthritis, do you find that drugs or other therapy provide little or no relief? Do you find that sometimes the drugs work and other times they don't? Do the medications make you ill in any way?

Variations in symptoms (present/absent, better/worse) are important, whether or not arthritis has been officially diagnosed. Do you have an increase or decrease in your pain, stiffness, swelling; inflammation in any joints; aching and/or tightness of muscles? Is your range of movement in any joint(s) better or worse

> at certain times of the day more than others?
> after certain meals?
> if you overeat or go on an eating binge?
> if you miss a meal?
> if you go on a fast?
> if you drink an alcoholic beverage?
> after an exposure to certain odors or fumes?
> in some locations more than in others (home, work, school, stores, vacation)?
> while engaged in certain nonathletic activities?
> at some times of year more than others?
> on some days of the week more than others?

If so, it may well be that some factor in your overall environment (food, beverages, airborne allergens, environmental chemicals) is triggering your flare-ups.

Do you have or have you ever had any of the other common forms of allergies? Do or did any close relatives suffer from hives, hay fever, eczema, asthma, and the like, or any other kind of allergic reactions? If so, it is possible that you are right to suspect that your aches, pains, swelling, and stiffness are manifestations of allergic arthritis—allergic reactions just as surely as are the stuffy, itchy, runny nose, sinusitis, coughing, wheezing, sneezing, red eyes, itching, hives, rash, headache, constipation, or diarrhea that physicians and the general public are more likely to associate with allergy.

You are well on your way to understanding—and, I sincerely hope, easing—your arthritis: a disorder that in 80 to 90 percent of the cases carefully studied to date by me and my fellow ecologists has been found to be an allergic-ecologic disorder of the joints, muscles, and other body structures. The addition of nutritional therapy to each person's comprehensive program of ecologic management will often benefit arthritic individuals, because their specific requirements for vitamins and minerals—their unique biochemical individuality—cannot be met by a "well-balanced diet." But first I wish to acquaint you with the major features of this painful, incapacitating, and at times crippling chronic disorder.

2

What Is Arthritis?

The Greek word for "joint" is *arthro,* and *itis* means "inflammation"—hence arthritis. Although, as we shall see, the disease takes many forms, in general it causes aching pain, stiffness, swelling, and often limitation of movement of one or more joints. Inflammation or erosion (or both) of the joints' inner structures, the ligaments that surround them, and nearby tendons and muscles creates the discomfort.

Arthritis primarily attacks synovial joints; these are the joints that have closed bursal sacs (also the sites of bursitis in other parts of the body) in which movement of the adjacent bones occurs. The fluid inside the bursal sac is called synovia, or synovial flud. As a joint is developing, two or more parts of the wall of the bursa become cartilage prior to birth, and in time these areas of cartilage become attached to the bones that come together (articulate) in the joint. The strands of fibrous tissue in the outer wall of the bursal sac blend with the fibrous tissue (periostium) that covers the outer surfaces of the bones, and the connective-tissue capsule of the joint is formed. Additional bands of connective tissue are formed in this area, and they are the ligaments that reinforce the joint-capsule wall and also help keep the ends of the articulating bones in position.

The following simplified drawings show some details of the development and structure of a typical joint. Look at them for a few minutes and it will be easier for you to understand the changes that occur in arthritis.

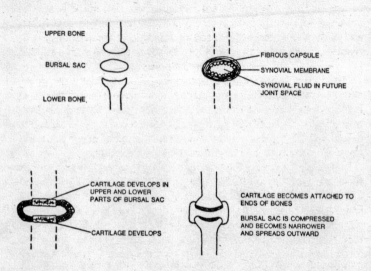

Arthritis can be excruciatingly painful. The usual prognosis is that it will become progressively worse. Patients often develop crippling deformities resulting in more and more severe limitations on bodily movement. And the frequent accompaniments of the disease—headache (often migraine), colitis, asthma, restlessness, fatigue, and depression, among others—bring additional discomfort to its sufferers. But the term *arthritis* encompasses several different disorders, which share many but not all symptoms.

Osteoarthritis

Osteoarthritis, also called degenerative joint disease, is the most common form of arthritis. It has been given the mistaken image of an "old-age disease," because it is the result of a wearing away of the cartilage in the joints, often due to many years of use. This erosion results in stiffness, and because it usually leaves behind a jagged area rather than a smooth surface, pain results that can be mild but is sometimes severe. Some degree of erosion is present in most elderly individuals and is generally accepted as an inherent part of the aging process. X-ray surveys in the United States and Great Britain indicate that 40 to 50 percent of the adult population have osteoarthritic changes in the hands or feet. It is estimated that 5 to 10 million Americans have symptoms due to these changes. But even this form of the "old-age disease" is not limited to the old: some people as young as forty (especially women) are afflicted with osteoarthritis, and as it often can be the result of improperly treated injuries or overuse, it can afflict anyone of any age who leads an active athletic life without taking appropriate precautions.

Osteoarthritis affects weight-bearing joints, especially the knees and hips. Although popularly referred to as osteoarthritis, this term is inaccurate because *itis* implies a disorder that is basically inflammatory, and this disease is in fact characterized by progressive deterioration of joint cartilage and the formation of dense bone and bony projections at the margins of the affected joints.

In its early stages the joint cartilage is softened and roughened; as the disease progresses, this cartilage may be destroyed. The exposed underlying bone no longer has its necessary protective cover of smooth cartilage that permits the articulating ends of the bones within the joint to glide smoothly over each other. The exposed, bared bone becomes more dense, and changes occur with the formation of new bone as the body tries to repair the local damage with regeneration of destroyed tissue.

The function of the relatively soft bone under the cartilage is to cushion the joint from the frequent mechanical stresses that result from the repeated impact of one bone against another during physical activities. With the passing of time, this softer shock-absorbing bone will have sustained numerous microscopic impact fractures that harden it. The reduced cushioning effect of the harder bone causes the initial damage to the overlying cartilage.

In addition to the aging process, there are local joint factors and a number of predisposing conditions that are important in the location and severity of the degeneration of joint cartilage. These include excessive wear and tear due to activities and occupation, injury, structural abnormalities, increased weight bearing with overweight, disorders of the cartilage, bleeding into the joint, and hereditary factors.

Rheumatoid Arthritis

Rheumatoid arthritis is described in medical textbooks as a chronic systemic disease of unknown cause for which there is no cure. It is characterized by inflammation of the joints, which is very often combined with other manifestations not directly associated with the joints. This disease occurs at all ages, including in young children, and is most often seen in young and middle-aged females. It is three times as common in females as in males and most often starts between the ages of forty and sixty.

Information from North America and Europe shows that rheumatoid arthritis affects at least 1 to 3 percent of the population. In the United States it is estimated that there are six million cases, one third of them people under fifty-five years of age. Among the young and middle-aged, it is the leading cause of occupational disability due to the high rate of serious interference with joint function.

The course of the disease varies greatly from patient to patient and is characterized by a striking tendency toward "spontaneous" remissions (temporary recovery) and exacerbations (flare-ups). 10 to 20 percent of arthritics will recover completely after their first attack. Between 30 and 50 percent of cases may be controlled with aspirin. Approximately 15 percent will be bed or wheelchair cases. The average patient will gradually become disabled and have increasing deformity.

In the majority of cases the onset is insidious, with general weakness, aching, and stiffness. This is gradually followed by joint inflammation with pain, swelling, redness, and tenderness. It usually starts in the small joints of the hands and feet and in most cases spreads to other areas, especially the wrists, elbows, hips, knees, and ankles. In severe cases almost all the joints may be affected, including the jaw, those between the spinal vertebrae, and even the joints in the larynx.

Many symptoms are not associated with the joints. There may be blood-vessel inflammation, chronic leg ulcers, anemia, enlarged lymph glands, and inflammation of the nerves (called neuritis), pericardium (area around the heart), sclerae (eyes), and lungs (inflammation and formation of nodules in the lung and pleura). In one out of twenty patients there is enlargement of the spleen.

The condition begins in the synovial membranes that line the joints. Inflammation of the synovial tissue leads to thickening of the joint lining and increase in the amount of fluid *(rheum)* in the joints. As inflammation of the synovia continues, the underlying cartilage at the ends of the bones is involved, and damage leads to erosion and destruction of the cartilage. The amount of disability, to a great extent, depends on the amount of damage done to the cartilage.

In severe cases large areas of bone may lose their cartilage, producing "raw spots" that may grow together with the formation of connective tissue (adhesions) between the denuded areas at the bone ends. The connective tissue matures and becomes stronger with calcium deposits and even the formation of new bone within the joint, leading to ankylosis (firm union between the bony surfaces) and interfering to different degrees with the motion of the joint, which may become fixed—totally immobile.

In other instances the loss of cartilage and bone within a joint and the weakening of supporting structures of the joint lead to the development of an unstable structure that involves some degree of dislocation of the bones from their normal positions. The skin, bones, and muscles adjacent to the joints may atrophy from disuse. Destruction can be rapid and severe in a small number of cases.

The traditional medical view of rheumatoid arthritis is that it is a chronic illness characterized by spontaneous remissions in most patients, who will, with varying degrees of restriction, be able to lead active lives with the use of medications that may (especially the cortisone/steroid drugs) cause more problems than the arthritis itself.

Patient and physician alike are educated not to expect a rapid resolution of the illness, and the outlook is "reasonably optimistic" that conservative treatment can relieve symptoms and keep disability to a minimum. No specific dietary measures or vitamin supplements are suggested, but weight reduction has a high priority in overweight arthritic patients. Associated depression may require psychological support from the attending physician, as well as sedatives or tranquilizers.

The basic program includes rest, medications to suppress inflammation and relieve pain, and physical therapy to preserve joint functions and maintain muscles. Some patients may require surgery.

This drug-oriented program of management may cover a long period of time and be associated with undesirable side effects. It is directed toward the suppression of symptoms, because there is no attention given to the detection and control of the specific identifiable cause(s) of most cases of the disease.

The drug of choice, part of basic conventional management, is aspirin or chemically related drugs known as salicylates. The chemical name for aspirin is acetylsalicylic acid. Salicylates may cause intestinal tract bleeding, dizziness, ringing in the ears (tinnitis), and other symptoms. It must be given with care to patients with stomach ulcers, bleeding tendencies, and asthma.

If the response to salicylates is not satisfactory after two months of treatment with rest and physical therapy, other anti-inflammatory drugs are employed. These are referred to as the nonaspirin NSAIDs—nonsteroidal (cortisonelike) antiinflammatory drugs. They have the same antiinflammatory activity as aspirin, but it is not possible to predict which drug will be effective in an individual patient. Each drug may have to be tried in a systematic sequence to determine which one will bring about the desired response. These drugs may be taken with aspirin or in place of aspirin.

There are two chemical groups of NSAIDs. The first group is derived from propionic acid and consists of Naprosyn (naproxen), Motrin (ibuprofen) and Nalfon (fenoprofen). The other family comes from indole: Indocin (indomethacin), Tolectin (tolmetin sodium), and Clinoril (sulindac). Many patients taking these NSAIDs will exhibit nervous-system toxicity, including headache and dizziness. Indocin has the greatest potential for gastrointestinal reactions.

Juvenile Rheumatoid Arthritis

Juvenile rheumatoid arthritis is a form of chronic arthritis in children that is also referred to as Still's disease, juvenile chronic polyarthritis, and juvenile chronic arthritis. It rarely begins before the age of one year, but it may start anytime after the first year. There are different types of juvenile rheumatoid arthritis that begin at different ages and more often in one sex or the other. It has been estimated that 5 percent of all cases of rheumatoid arthritis begin before the age of sixteen.

Juvenile rheumatoid arthritis (JRA) is defined as the onset of the disease under age sixteen. It has some features that distinguish it from rheumatoid arthritis (RA) in adults. These clinical differences include high fever, rash, high white blood cell count, eye involvement, growth disturbances, and increased tendency to have the disease localize in a single joint. In about 20 percent of cases the onset is acute and rapidly progressing, with general symptoms of illness such as fever and rash associated with enlargement of the spleen and inflammation of the pericardial sac around the heart, and in some cases these manifestations may be present for several weeks before the joint inflammation is evident.

In one third of these cases the disease begins in a single joint (monoarticular), and in half the cases the onset resembles adult RA and includes more than one joint (polyarticular). Pauciarticular JRA involves only a few joints and may affect the eyes. Skeletal growth in bones adjacent to inflamed joints may be either accelerated or retarded. If the heart is affected, the illness may be confused with acute rheumatic fever, but JRA frequently begins before age five, the joint symptoms do not migrate from joint to joint, the vertebrae in the neck are involved, the white blood cells are markedly increased, and rash frequently occurs.

The synovial tissue lining the joints becomes inflamed and the synovitis may last for weeks, months, or years. If the synovitis persists for a long enough period of time, the cartilage at the ends of the bones within the joint and the bone underlying the cartilage may be damaged. The cartilage may not regenerate at all, although it does have slight regenerative properties. Damage to the ligaments and tendons surrounding joints may also occur. Permanent joint damage occurs because the bones may be dislocated or fused together, tissue may be destroyed, and muscles and other structures surrounding the joint may shorten (contractures), causing deformities in the absence of damage within the joints. These serious complications do not occur often, and most children do not sustain permanent joint damage or deformity.

The diagnosis is based solely on the presence of the characteristic clinical findings and the careful exclusion of other conditions that also are associated with arthritis and joint pains. Destructive joint changes occurring late in severe cases of the disease will be noted in X-rays, but there are no other specific diagnostic tests that establish the diagnosis.

Complete remission occurs in 50 percent or more of the children with JRA. The major consequences of this illness are permanently restricted joint function, heart disease, and chronic eye inflammation.

At least 75 percent of the children who have JRA will recover from their illness without having any important residual disability if they are given what is generally accepted as proper care during active periods of their illness. Currently approved methods of treatment are symptomatic—directed against the symptoms of the disease—and not curative. This is because the underlying factors responsible for JRA are poorly understood.

Treatment of this chronic illness consists of medication, physical and occupational therapy, psychological reinforcement (to offset the discouraging aspects of JRA), and surgery (to reconstruct joint damage). Education and counseling are important because the affected child's needs and limitations may have a great impact on family activities and the uncertainty of the diagnosis and prognosis cause severe psychological stress for everyone concerned.

Although cortisone-related (steroid) drugs such as Prednisone can often work magic in this illness, their use must be limited to the severe manifestations that do not respond to aspirin and other nonsteroid drugs. The possibility of cardiac damage and loss of vision require careful medical supervision. Another serious problem associated with steroid therapy is that steroids cause growth retardation, and although they may be necessary in the management of this illness, they may augment the growth retardation that is a natural feature of JRA.

It is not within the scope of this book for me to review the five different forms of this disease that can usually be distinguished from each other within six months after its onset. It is even possible that what we call JRA is more than one disease. If your child is among the estimated 250,000 cases in the United States, the specialist you consult will review this matter with you in depth, since each type of the illness has certain physical and laboratory characteristics, follows a particular course, affects more girls than boys or vice versa, and is associated with different kinds of complications.

I have not had any personal experience in the care of children with acute JRA during the past thirty years. On the other hand, my technicians and I have performed symptom-duplicating provocative tests that have reproduced familiar muscle and joint pains in children, which indicates that allergies or allergylike sensitivities do involve these structures in childhood, even though these children did not have a confirmed diagnosis of JRA or a suspicious medical history.

As far as I know, none of my fellow ecologists has had an opportunity to study the ecologic-allergic aspects of JRA in more than a few children from the onset of their illness. The small number of cases I have learned about from other clinical ecologists involved reports on children who were seen during the chronic phase of their illness—after their acute symptoms cleared, if the onset of the illness was characterized by systemic manifestations. The investigation of JRA cases established the fact that foods and chemicals were important factors in the genesis of JRA. They reported that ecologic management based on measures to control the exposure to JRA-related factors by diet and environmental changes and precautions were very effective in controlling this illness.

Lupus (Systemic Lupus Erythematosis—SLE)

Systemic lupus erythematosis is a chronic inflammatory disease, similar in some ways to rheumatoid arthritis, that may develop at any period of life but most often affects women between the ages of ten and forty years. It exists in many forms ranging from very mild to severe and even fatal. Each year there are six thousand to twelve thousand new cases in the United States alone. SLE may affect various parts of the body singly or in combination. Among the structures involved are the skin, joints, kidneys, nervous system, linings of body cavities, and other organs. There is a striking tendency toward remissions and exacerbations, and laboratory abnormalities are frequently found in the blood.

There are two types of the illness: systemic and discoid. Discoid is a disorder that is usually limited to the skin and usually confined to a facial rash that may be similar to that which occurs in SLE. Less than 5 percent of the cases of discoid lupus erythematosis will include involvement of other organs and structures besides the skin.

SLE occasionally includes a butterfly-shape facial reddening over the bridge of the nose and the cheeks. Other findings in SLE may be discoid lupus, Reynaud's phenomenon (pallor caused by spasm of small arteries that reduce the blood flow), photosensitivity, nondeforming arthritis, kidney inflammation, pericarditis (inflammation of the sac that encloses the heart), pleurisy, and nervous system involvement (psychotic behavior or convulsions). The general symptoms that usually appear first are fever, weakness, easy fatigue, and loss of weight. The majority of cases develop anemia because the red blood cells are destroyed and there are decreased numbers of white blood cells and abnormal bleeding, as well as other changes in the blood (these can cause false positive blood tests for syphilis in as many as one out of five cases of SLE).

The treatment of SLE is directed toward protection of vital organs by reducing or controlling inflammation. Aspirin is used to reduce fever and relieve pain, especially when the joints are affected. Milder forms are treated with certain antimalaria drugs. Sterioids are given in most cases to reduce the inflammation in acute crises.

The course of the illness varies but very often becomes chronic and smolders on for months and years, with ups and downs. There may be very long symptom-free periods. The major factor with regard to survival is the severity of the kidney disorder and the response of the kidney to treatment. Cases involving mainly the joints do best.

Other Forms

Bursitis is the painful inflammation of a bursa. Bursae are synovial-fluid-containing sacs that reduce local friction between bones, muscles, tendons, and ligaments. The most frequent cause of bursitis is a local injury. The bursae most commonly affected are located in the shoulders, hips, elbows, and knees.

Ankylosing spondylitis (AS) is a disease of the joints in the spine, the sacroiliac joints in the lower back, and the tissues next to the vertebrae. AS affects eight males to every female and is a common cause of low back pain and stiffness in young men that usually begins insidiously between the ages of ten and thirty years. It affected one individual out of two thousand in a survey conducted in England.

Approximately 25 percent of the patients develop a serious inflammation of some internal parts of the eyes, and the aorta (the large blood vessel that carries blood from the heart to supply the entire body with oxygen, food, etc.) may also become inflamed, leaving a damaged aortic heart valve where the aorta is connected to the heart. The tissue changes in the lower back may seriously affect the nerves of the end of the spinal cord in a few individuals and cause local pain or loss of sensation and loss of control of the bladder and rectum.

A third to half of the patients with this condition, also known as Marie-Strumpell Spondylitis or rheumatoid spondylitis, have inflammation in other joints, especially the hips and shoulders. The outstanding feature of this disease is deposition of calcium, bone formation in the ligaments of the spine, and gradual development of a poker-back deformity of the spine. Treatment is directed toward prevention of spinal deformity as well as suppressing inflammation and relieving pain.

Gout is a complex group of diseases that are caused by an excess of uric acid in the body. Gout has a strong hereditary trait—high levels of uric acid are found in the blood in 15 to 25 percent of close relatives of patients with gout. Uric acid dissolved in the blood causes no problems, but it causes gout when it is precipitated as sodium urate in tissues throughout the body.

In the joints sodium urate causes an acute inflammation that is extremely painful. Acute gouty arthritis occurs primarily in the feet and ankles and occasionally the knees. The tissues around the joint and the nearby skin may be severely inflamed with redness, extreme swelling, and marked tenderness that often seem to suggest the presence of an infection. Gout in its various forms afflicts about 1½ million Americans, most of them men.

There are other, less common forms of arthritis, and there is also joint pain that is *not* arthritis. Circulatory problems, infections, stress, or referred pain from other parts of the body can produce arthritislike symptoms, but most of the cases of true arthritis can be diagnosed by blood tests or tests of synovial fluid obtained by aspirating joint fluid. *Rheumatism* is a word some people use for arthritis. It's not a formal disease, however, but a term used to describe those aches, pains, and stiff feelings that beset all of us sometimes.

Some forms of arthritis seem to have a hereditary factory: they run in families. Many allergies and environmental sensitivities run in families, too.

It has been speculated that a virus might be the culprit, but that has never been proved. The symptoms associated with many allergic reactions resemble virus infections, too.

Various theories have blamed the inappropriate leakage of enzymes or microbes through blood-vessel walls into joints that become arthritic. The leakage of fluid through allergen-affected blood-vessel walls is characteristic of many allergic responses, too.

It has been noted that some forms of arthritis begin or flare up at times of emotional stress, though it is not known why. Many allergic people are more sensitive during times of stress, too.

So far, despite the vast sums spent on research, about the only thing that conventional modern medicine claims to be sure about arthritis is that the cause is unknown. My fellow ecologists and I thoroughly disagree with this point of view, since we have repeatedly turned this disease on and off by challenges with and elimination of arthritis-inducing environmental substances that we have identified through our special testing methods.

One aspect of the disease that particularly puzzles researchers is the group of apparently unrelated disorders that often accompany arthritis. After all, why should headaches, colitis, asthma, fatigue, depression, or rashes occur along with a disorder of the joints? Of interest to the bioecologists (who also do not claim to understand with certainty the basic cause of the disease) is the fact that these arthritis-associated conditions in other systems are common, body-wide allergic reactions. I view arthritis as one aspect of a systemic allergic or allergylike disorder that affects many organs. In a majority of cases arthritis consists of the joint and muscle reactions to specific, identifiable environmental substances that are also affecting many other body structures. These offending agents reach allergically reactive sites throughout the body via the bloodstream, after gaining entrance to the body through the digestive tract and/or the lungs.

3

Standard Treatments for Arthritis

Arthritis has been a recognized disease for over two thousand five hundred years, since the time of Hippocrates, the founder of modern medicine. Archeological evidence indicates that it afflicted people of prehistoric times as well. Over the centuries and well into current times, sufferers and their physicians have tried a wide variety of remedies for arthritis—copper bracelets, kelp, vinegar, mussel essence, and devil's claw root, as well as many drugs.

Some of these treatments, even the most apparently bizarre, seem to have relieved arthritis symptoms for some people, and others have proved effective for other individuals, while many have been ineffective or harmful. Today arthritis therapy is clothed in more scientific garb, but its effects vary as widely as those of previous generations. No therapy is foolproof, and many drugs and procedures are associated with undesirable side effects.

In fact, as you may know if you've ever visited a rheumatologist or other physician because of symptoms of arthritis, doctors freely admit that they know of no cure for your disease. Instead, the doctor may offer consolation and the reassurance that with rest; hot baths; physiotherapy; following a prescribed exercise program; use of one of several drugs that are employed to control pain, inflammation, and muscle spasm; and frequent office visits; the symptoms can usually be controlled. As time goes on, if you are like many arthritic patients, you will be given doctor-supervised doses of any or all of the following medicines, separately or in combination.

Aspirin, for example, is the most widely prescribed arthritis medication. Taken daily usually in very large doses, it often relieves joint and muscle pain and reduces the inflammation that causes pain and stiffness. The dosage, however, must be determined by a physician, and although it helps most people, it does not bring relief to all. In addition, aspirin is regarded as the safest drug available for arthritis treatment, but it often has unpleasant and at times serious side effects, including gastrointestinal bleeding and ringing in the ears. It is the least expensive of the various treatments—the large daily doses required cost approximately ten dollars a month—but a physician's continuing supervision is required, and those fees add to the cost of the therapy.

Other treatments for the symptoms of arthritis (and remember, these are only symptomatic treatments; not even the most modern drug therapies are *cures*) carry the danger of even more serious hazards with them.

Corticosteroids are a related group of potent antiinflammatory drugs that are administered to arthritics if more conservative treatment fails. For many they can dramatically reduce joint inflammation, but prednisone and the other cortisonelike steroid medications such as prednisolone, triamcinolone, methylprednisolone, dexamethasone, betamethasone, and paramethasone have frequent and potentially life threatening complications. They suppress inflammation, but they do not correct the underlying process. They lead to fluid retention, obesity, stomach problems (peptic ulcers), and skin trouble, and they may aggravate latent diabetes and psychic disorders. They interfere with and can greatly complicate the treatment of other conditions, including certain infections and fractures. They also decrease the steroid-treated individual's ability to respond adequately to serious stress associated with injuries, surgery, and infections.

When steroids are injected directly into a painful arthritic joint, the dangers to other organs or systems are minimal and the benefits may be great—but only for a short time and not in every case. This treatment cannot be given too frequently, since steroids may have harmful effects on the cartilage within the injected joint.

Because of the hazards of the corticosteroids, a new series of nonsteroidal antiinflammatory drugs—*NSAIDs*—has been developed. These drugs, which include indomethacin, fenoprofen, naproxen, and ibuprofen, have fewer side effects than steroids, and they relieve fever (antipyretic) and pain (analgesic). They are only about as beneficial as aspirin and cost considerably more.

Phenylbutazone (Butazolidan) is a good antiinflammatory agent that, unfortunately, is associated with dangerous toxic effects and should not be used without close supervision. The drug can damage the bone marrow (which produces blood cells) and cause exfoliative dermatitis, a serious skin condition.

Penicillamine is another antiarthritis medication that is so toxic that it is administered only to those whose chronic rheumatoid arthritis is very severe and has not responded to other treatment, because it can damage the kidneys and the bone-marrow tissues that produce our blood cells. In fact, it is still considered to be an experimental drug for the treatment of arthritis.

Another family of experimental pharmaceuticals used to treat arthritis, the *immunosuppressive* or cytotoxic drugs, was developed to treat cancer and assist in the "taking" of transplanted organs (*cytotoxic* means "toxic to cells"). These anticancer chemotherapeutic compounds include cyclophosphamide, methotrexate, chlorambucil and azathioprine. These very dangerous drugs suppress the body's immune system, which may become overactive in some forms of arthritis and thereby play a role in joint inflammation. The body needs its immune system's protective powers to defend against other illnesses, and immunosuppressives must be used very carefully and only in extreme and stubborn cases.

Injections of *gold salts,* such as sodium aurothiomalate (Myochrisine) and aurothioglucose (Solganal) may sound like a somewhat exotic form of treatment, but they actually are a traditional, tried-and-true technique that has been used for fifty years. They bring relief to some sufferers of rheumatoid arthritis by increasing the likelihood of a remission in an unknown manner. Gold treatment is known as chrysotherapy. Some specialists start gold treatment in the early stages of the disease, but others use it only in cases that do not respond after several months or more conservative treatment. It helps about two thirds of rheumatoid arthritics but produces both unpleasant side effects and serious complications in the skin, oral cavity, kidneys, and blood. Its benefits and hazards take several months to show up, and it is quite expensive.

Antimalarial drugs such as chloroquine and hydroxychloroquine are occasionally employed in the treatment of RA and lupus. Related to quinine, which is used in treating malaria, they have a moderate effect on joint inflammation, but they are not used as often as in the past because they carry the risk of blindness that occasionally results from irreversible damage to the retina.

Among the newer "discoveries" in the field of arthritis treatment are *total lymphoid radiation, acupuncture,* and topical *DMSO.* Radiation therapy of the lymphatic system has recently been used as a last resort in patients suffering from extremely painful and crippling arthritis. It is expensive, makes the patients nauseous and tired, and causes hair loss; it has a particularly dangerous side effect—radiation-related cancers.

DMSO, or dimethylsulfoxide, is a substance arthritics rub onto affected joints that often produces great relief. The United States government, however, has approved it only for use by veterinarians, so it remains controversial; and it does not help all who try it.

Acupuncture, the ancient Oriental technique of inserting small needles at various points of the body, also relieves the pain that many arthritics suffer, but it, too, is a controversial and often expensive treatment that is little understood and that does not help all patients.

If swelling and inflammation continue to have prolonged, serious effects on your joints, *surgery* may be "the only answer." Surgery is used in many thousands of arthritis cases to remove the troublesome synovial membranes (see page 41), to cut away overgrown bone, or to replace damaged joints with synthetic devices. The problem with such surgery, aside from the hazards that any major operation poses, is that it cannot cure arthritis or prevent its recurrence in other joints, any more than can all the other forms of treatment.

So what do we have so far? When you go to a physician for relief of arthritis pain, you *may* get just that—relief, if only temporary, by taking one or a combination of costly and potentially dangerous drugs whose function is little understood. Or you may get little or no relief, if your arthritis does not respond to traditional drug therapies, as many sufferers have unfortunately discovered.

Established medicine has found no specific demonstrable cause, no cure, no preventive measure to stop further flare-ups of arthritis. In addition, traditional medicine has not found any form of symptom relief that is both safe and effective for all patients. The pharmaceutical industry has to date succeeded only in discovering new drugs for treatments that require continuing, close medical supervision with laboratory studies to detect undesirable side effects early.

When all else fails, the best your doctor may be able to suggest is a combination of symptom-relieving treatments consisting of heat, hydrotherapy, rest, exercise, and, as a last resort, more dangerous drugs, blood cleansing (plasmapheresis), or surgery that may temporarily ease the discomfort enough to "live with" the arthritis—which is just the way folks have lived with "the rheumatiz" for generations.

Recently the medical schools of Harvard and Stanford universities reported on their investigation of "Total Lymphoid Radiation," moderately strong X-ray treatments for "intractable rheumatoid arthritis." Before the radiation treatment was considered, many of the arthritic patients had been unsuccessfully treated with very potent cytotoxic or poisonous drugs—cyclophosphamide and azathioprine, which are administered with extreme caution to very carefully selected patients.

The preliminary trials of this radiation treatment were reported as "effective in reducing joint inflammation," and "all patients experienced nausea, anorexia (loss of appetite) and fatigue as a result of irradiation," which is almost always associated with reversible hair loss. "In contrast to the Stanford study, disease activity returned in the Boston patients after about one year rather than eighteen months." In other words, after a single course of potentially dangerous X-ray treatments (costing about $5,000) that might very well lead to serious future complications, the patients relapsed.

Both studies were reported to the medical profession in the prestigious *New England Journal of Medicine* and were referred to as having "come up with an extremely interesting finding" by H. C. Neu, M.D., of the editorial staff of *Infectious Diseases,* published in January 1982.*

One patient for whom the radiation treatment had been prescribed came to me for an evaluation instead. Her trip to my office in Connecticut was sponsored by a Canadian Lions Club whose members had become aware of her serious arthritic condition. Her condition had not responded to any standard or advanced form of current medical treatment—including an $18,000 series of immunologic plasmapheresis treatments.

At age twenty-six Anne had been informed that the only remaining hope was the series of X-ray treatments that would provide total lymphoid irradiation. As noted, this treatment causes nausea, loss of appetite and hair, and has the very real danger of causing cancer to develop in the patient twenty years later. This threat might not be a serious problem for the elderly (who would probably not expect to live long enough to suffer from this side effect), but for someone Anne's age this is a severe risk to take. And balancing this risk is

---

*Strober and Kaplan (305:969, 1981) Stanford Group. Trentham and Austen (305:976, 1981) Harvard Group. *New England Journal of Medicine.*

only the promise of a possible twelve- to eighteen-month remission of the arthritis. Anne wisely refused the treatment.

Our consultation was most enlightening with regard to the course of her severe childhood arthritis, hospitalizations, and numerous drug reactions. After a period of remission she had married a young man who moved his upholstery business into their home, with all the attendant synthetic materials, lumber, glues, stains, paint-stripping compounds, and finishes of his trade, which polluted the entire home with chemical agents. There were many other important diagnostic clues in her history, and when they were explored by my laboratory technicians, we learned enough about her arthritis to begin effective treatment. We did not use drugs. Instead we identified the rather easy-to-find causes of her unrecognized *allergic* illness.

She is currently receiving desensitizing injections to control her allergic reactions to airborne allergens such as dust, molds, and pollens. She is also following an individualized Rotary Diversified Diet that excludes those foods we discovered she is allergic to and properly spaces her exposure to other foods so they will not build up in her system and cause a cumulative reaction. As a result of these measures, Anne's arthritis has already abated markedly. Soon we hope to have the upholstery business and its associated chemical pollutants removed from her home, along with other biologically active chemical substances to which she is susceptible.

I am not writing to criticize the sincere efforts of the dedicated, tireless physicians who are engaged in this research. Their objective deserves nothing but our respect and admiration. They were seeking a way to bring relief from a terrible, painful, and crippling disease. But I am frustrated and very much concerned about this situation, as are other ecologists and our colleagues in clinical nutrition. Look at the many failures of the modern miracle drugs that brought these arthritis victims to cytotoxic drugs and radiation. Could simple, conservative ecologic management have prevented this medical tragedy? Isn't it time to pause and reflect about what is going on out there in our modern "superscience" approach to illness, which ignores the already demonstrated superiority of the ecologic cause-and-effect diagnosis and cause-directed treatments that are in harmony with common sense and nature?

The cost and lack of complete effectiveness of the widely employed, medically recognized arthritis-relief techniques are major reasons why so many people turn to self-remedies and informal folk medicine. Some folk remedies people have sworn by for years but which modern-day doctors abhor include drinking vinegar, eating honey, and using snake venom.

Some arthritics say that they find relief in warm, dry climates, although weather conditions do not affect all sufferers. Recent medical research has found that climate has an impact on arthritis symptoms when humidity is high and the barometric pressure is low.

Some arthritics have reported that changes in their diets have improved their arthritis. During one of my recent public lectures, a woman told me that her grandfather's arthritis cleared up completely when he stopped drinking milk and eating milk products. It is not unusual for me or my colleagues to be given this type of report. Traditionally oriented nutritionists and the medical establishment state that they have found no connection between diet and arthritis. I can only conclude that this situation exists because they have never looked for the connection. They do agree that the popular but nebulous entity "good nutrition" is important for arthritics just as for everyone else.

One bit of folk wisdom that was unknown to me until I participated in a radio talk show in Vermont is based on the well-established and very often effective (but not generally employed) ecologic technique of therapeutic fasting. A woman caller to the show asked me if it really was possible to cure this disease by the folk method of "starving the arthritis," and I answered yes. You will learn that this is true for many food-allergic individuals who have allergically reactive joints that clear up as if by magic after a four- to six-day fast. In fact, we now have found scientific explanations for the success of some of the old-fashioned folk-remedies and substances used by the medicine men and priests of other cultures. The use of quinine from tree bark, cocaine from coca leaves, digitalis from foxglove, morphine from poppies, and penicillin from bread mold are some of them.

What is of special interest to the clinical ecologists, whether we are looking at "folk remedies" or "scientific treatments," is that some therapies do help one individual and not another, or that an exposure to some environmental substance may provoke minor discomfort or harmful effects in one person and not another. For us those facts, pointing to very important individual biologic differences in responses to environmental exposures (biochemical individuality*), offer clues to the allergic or allergylike nature of arthritis and numerous other conditions.

Avoidance of a given food or foods that specifically affect their joints as well as other body structures will help many arthritic

---

*Biochemical individuality is a brilliant concept discovered and developed by Roger J. Williams, Ph.D., a world authority and distinguished researcher in the field of nutrition.

individuals who are sensitive to these particular offending dietary substances. Complete elimination of the same food or group of foods cannot possibly relieve all allergic arthritis sufferers, since they do not have exactly the same pattern of food allergies, and one elimination diet cannot possibly be effective in all cases.

Arthritis is what I call a patient-specific syndrome. This means that every biologically unique arthritic patient has his or her own one-of-a-kind body chemistry and immune system, which determine his or her particular allergic responses. Tearing up one's roots, leaving family, friends, and a good job in order to move to a new climate, may simply remove a particular allergic-arthritic individual from an ecologically bad place to an ecologically good place that happens to be free from the specific environmental substances that trigger the symptoms. An ecologically undiagnosed arthritic who is allergically reactive to foods, inhalants, and various environmental chemical substances will not find relief in a new climate because he or she will continue to eat unsuspected food offenders and will still be exposed to all the potential chemical offenders that are associated with modern living.

In some cases just moving across the street, around the corner, or to another part of town might be the answer. Perhaps changing methods of housecleaning or place of work or occupation in the same city will be all that is necessary to gain relief from arthritis that is caused by various chemical substances or airborne allergens present in a specific building. An expensive long-distance move could be undertaken unnecessarily because of modern medicine's complete failure to recognize a case of chemically susceptible arthritis that is set off by avoidable indoor air pollution, or to spot a sufferer from inhalant mold allergy with arthritic manifestations who only needed to remove mold-containing potted plants or correct a mildew condition in the living quarters, basement, or crawl space.

Rather than following the traditional method of trying one form of drug therapy after another on a patient, the clinical ecologist is usually able to determine in advance which measure or combination of measures will be effective. This is because we have discovered and confirmed that 80 to 90 percent of all arthritis is a musculoskeletal manifestation of an often bodywide (systemic) allergic or allergy-like reaction to some substances in the diet or the environment that affect the joints and surrounding structures as well as the muscles. Our treatment is directed against the specific causes, not the symptoms. Not only can the bioecologic approach relieve arthritis symptoms and often lead to reversal of tissue damage, but in the long run it can prevent recurrence of those symptoms and block the often crippling damage that results from continuous or recurrent joint inflammation.

4

What Is "Allergy"?

In order to understand how bioecologic medicine can help arthritis, it is necessary for me to explain further what we ecologists mean by the term *allergy,* which we use in its broadest, original definition, when we discuss the numerous physical and mental disorders that result when susceptible people react to a variety of common substances they frequently come in contact with during the course of normal daily activities. Some of these daily activities are essential to the maintenance of life itself. Eating, drinking, and breathing are the life-sustaining processes responsible for an unending series of exposures to numerous substances in our environment that enter the body by way of the digestive and respiratory tracts.

For many people "having an allergy" means getting the sneezes, sniffles, and red, itching, watery eyes when certain pollens or dandruff (dander) from house pets is in the air. For others it means becoming short of breath, with rapid breathing, coughing, and asthmatic wheezing after eating certain foods or after inhaling house dust or particles of many kinds of molds or mildew that are in the air, or breaking out all over with very itchy mosquito-bitelike hives, with puffy eyelids and lips, after eating such foods as tomato, egg, fish, or strawberries. Those are examples of some of the common allergic reactions, but "having an allergy" means far more than that.

My colleagues and I in ecologic medicine have proven that allergy, or allergylike sensitivity, to substances we eat, drink, breathe, and otherwise absorb into our bodies can be the result of environmental factors that cause a very large and diverse group of often serious physical and mental-emotional-behavioral ailments from migraine to mental illness, from chronic fatigue to compulsive eating (obesity) and drinking (alcoholism), from insomnia to hyperactivity and irritability, depression, and many other conditions such as colitis, ulcers, abdominal pain, bloating, indigestion, constipation, diarrhea, gallbladder colic, growing pains, bed-wetting and other urinary tract disorders, hypertension, confusion, mood swings, impaired concentration, short attention span, nervousness, dizzy spells, disorientation, learning disabilities, and so on.

I have described and thoroughly discussed the enormous scope of allergic-ecologic disorders of the mind and body in my previous book, *Dr. Mandell's Five-Day Allergy Relief System,* and you will also be able to read comprehensive reports and enlightening discussions of our studies in the books and other publications listed on pages 261–263.

The following relatively simple basic concepts and discoveries will enable you to understand the connection between allergy and arthritis. Think of your body as a beautifully designed and fantastically complex chemical reactor. At any given moment thousands of interrelated, life-sustaining biochemical reactions are taking place in and on the surfaces of the billions of cells that your body is made of. Chemical reactions also occur in the extracellular fluid that comes from your blood plasma through the walls of the capillaries and surrounds these cells, bringing nutrients and removing wastes. Every activity that takes place within this wonderful mechanism of your multiple-system body, from digestion to thought, occurs as a result of some simple or complex chain (pathway or sequence) of highly organized, indispensable, enzyme-regulated biochemical reactions.

Your body is composed of and is surrounded by a world consisting of thousands of simple and complex chemicals. Everything you eat, drink, breathe, or touch is a chemical substance that may contain other chemicals that have been added to or contaminate them, and all of them react in one way or another during the unending cycles of metabolism within the extremely complicated chemistry of your body.

This biochemical and structural masterpiece—your body—is also an independent, mobile, self-regulating, living unit; a magnificently functioning, highly integrated package, if you like. You may be accustomed to thinking of yourself as a collection of systems or small "packages": nervous system, respiratory system, cardiovascular system, digestive system, and so forth. On the other hand, you may see yourself as body, mind, perceptions, emotions, and spirit. It is important that you understand that each part of the human body, including the brain and its psyche, is connected with every other part in many ways, with nerves and tissue-regulating hormones for "communication" and blood vessels for "transportation" and cellular exchange of nutrients, by-products, and wastes.

Because of this complex interrelationship, what enters any area of the total system can affect any or all the other areas. If you breathe in some house-dust particles, mold spores, or ragweed pollen, or if you inhale tobacco smoke, fumes of mothballs, fresh paint, or automobile exhaust, they may produce an immediate "contact-surface" reaction in the form of coughing, sneezing, wheezing, or irritation of the nose, throat, and bronchial tubes as they affect the allergically reactive cells present in people with respiratory-tract allergy. When they are swallowed or inhaled, these airborne particles and chemical fumes are also capable of causing extreme difficulty in the form of internal symptoms, because they can reach and affect your entire body.

Inhaled airborne particles that are present indoors (dust, dust motes, animal dander, or molds) or outdoors (trees, grass or weed pollens, molds, animal dander, or scales and other tiny parts of insects) can cause internal (systemic) changes in at least three ways.

1. They become trapped in the moist, sticky mucus in the nose and throat, and some allergically active substances can dissolve in the moisture and pass through the walls of the membranes lining the upper respiratory tract and soon enter the circulation for bodywide distribution.
2. Animal research with radioactive material has demonstrated that some active substances reach the brain directly from the oral cavity by an as-yet-unidentified route.
3. Allergen-containing mucus that is swallowed enters the upper part of the digestive system by way of the stomach and undergoes the same processing that ingested foods are subjected to. Eventually the allergically or biologically active components of the digested airborne allergens pass through the walls of the intestines and enter the minute intestinal blood vessels (capillaries), which come together like the tributaries of a river, becoming

veins that transport substances from the intestine to the liver for processing by the liver cells. Then blood from the liver goes directly to the heart, which pumps the allergen-containing blood throughout the entire circulatory system. The allergens reach every allergically reactive cell in every organ of the body, and this certainly includes the muscles and joints and nearby structures that are the tissues involved in cases of arthritis.

In addition, the air-polluting chemical fumes present in indoor and outdoor air accompany the atmospheric oxygen we need as it passes through the walls of the capillary blood vessels in the lungs and enters the circulation. Along with our oxygen, these highly reactive fumes reach all the active and potential arthritis sites throughout the entire body.

I have given my readers this detailed information because it is very important that you fully understand how arthritis flares up as pollens and molds appear in the environment and build up to seasonal peaks during particular times of the year. And you now understand why allergylike sensitivity to chemically derived substances (chemical susceptibility) such as petroleum and coal-tar products, and the natural gas or fuel oil in your home as well as manufactured pollutants like tobacco smoke, paint, mothballs, hair spray, air fresheners, disinfectants, perfume, and the like can be important factors in the causation of arthritis as well as of many other conditions throughout the body.

This explains how a certain food can make a child hyperactive; why stove gas can make the cook and everyone else in the family tired, depressed, restless, or irritable at mealtimes; why the fumes of freshly applied paint can produce headaches, confusion, and/or nausea—and why any of a number of substances in the environment can cause arthritis. It also explains why a person with arthritis may also suffer from colitis, migraine headaches, asthma, fatigue, itching, and bladder symptoms. It would be such a blessing to hundreds of thousands of patients if their physicians at last were to realize that these disorders do not just happen to occur in a single body by coincidence and that these associated body-wide conditions are not an unrelated assortment of psychosomatic/neurotic/hypochondriac reactions. With an ecologic orientation this complicated and confusing group of coexisting diseases could easily be recognized and successfully managed or at least significantly improved by any physician who makes the necessary effort to become familiar with the genesis, diagnosis, and treatment of multiple-system allergies to commonly encountered substances in the environment.

The arthritic reaction to an allergic substance is not difficult to understand once you have a clear picture of the basic cellular mechanisms involved in any allergic or allergylike response.

No matter what substance causes an allergic type of reaction or where in the body it occurs, the underlying mechanism of the interaction is essentially the same. When the walls of the delicate, one-cell-thick capillaries—microscopic blood vessels that transfer substances between the blood and the fluids that surround the cells (from the main blood vessel channels to the tissues in our organs)—encounter a substance to which they are allergically sensitive, they become more permeable. The openings between the cells become larger, and in this abnormal state, the temporarily damaged capillaries leak an increased amount of fluid from the blood plasma into the tissues they serve, causing congestion.

You have already observed this kind of reaction in the skin after someone has been bitten by a mosquito. The affected skin becomes edematous (swollen) because the capillaries injured by mosquito saliva in the area surrounding the bite have leaked fluid from the blood into the skin more rapidly than it can be reabsorbed. This process is part of the body's self-protection system, the immune system. When something that is potentially dangerous enters the system—as in the form of a toxin or the bacteria or viruses contained in a vaccine—the body reacts by diluting the offending substance and rushing protective cells and special elements in the blood to the area to fight off the foreign invader, and this immunologic "battle" creates the swelling and inflammation associated with insect bites or immunizing shots or infections.

In addition to changes in the walls of the capillary blood vessels that permit edema fluid to leak into the surrounding tissues, there are two other easily recognized allergic reacitons that all of us are familiar with. Smooth muscles that are not under our voluntary control accomplish many functions when their fibers contract or shorten. The smooth muscles present in tubular (pipelike) structures of the body control the diameter of these structures and make it easier or harder for substances to flow through them.

In asthma there is too much contraction or spasm of the smooth muscles that form rings that encircle the small bronchial tubes deep in the lungs. Contraction of these muscles will decrease the diameter of these passageways and reduce the flow of air entering the numerous microscopic air sacs that transfer oxygen from the air to the blood and restrict the airflow back out of the chest. This allergic bronchial muscle spasm causes shortness of breath, and wheezing sounds are noted as air travels through the narrowed bronchial tubes. Until the causes of this spasm are identified and controlled, medications are employed to relieve this spasm.

Unfortunately some physicians do not "believe" in allergy and do not refer their patients to allergists whose diagnostic studies will usually identify the cause of the asthma. Without knowledge of the causes of the patient's bronchial allergy, the nonbelieving physician cannot eliminate or control the responsible factors because he does not know what they are. His care is limited to the use of emergency treatments and the prescription of daily symptom-suppressing medications that cannot cure the illness.

As long as the drugs are taken, the undiagnosed (with respect to underlying cause) allergic symptoms may be partially or well controlled, but nothing else has been done for the long-term benefit of the asthmatic patient. The illness is always "present," because the unidentified causes continue to operate under cover of the anti-asthma drugs. The illness remains in a latent, ready-to-flare-up state that will in most cases produce symptoms within a few hours after the symptom-suppressing medications are discontinued.

If medications are not very effective in a complex case of asthma—and the situation is not uncommon—the patient may be blamed directly or indirectly by drug- and psychiatrically oriented physicians because they really do not know how to diagnose many of the asthmatic patients they see. And they have a number of comforting self-deceptions to fall back on. "This is a case of 'intrinsic' asthma, in which there are no external physical causes to be identified." "This is a psychosomatic disorder due to the stress of unidentified emotional factors that the asthmatic patient cannot cope with." Or, "The patient has a treatment-refractory (resistant) condition." This last explanation blames the patient for not getting better, instead of the physician whose inappropriate treatment cannot succeed. If the environmental allergic factors are not suspected and searched for, these causes are not going to be detected. It is obvious that without this vital information, it is not possible to prescribe the correct diet, initiate or properly formulate desensitizing injection treatments, or institute the necessary environmental changes that will directly attack the root of the problem.

If the reader substitutes the word *arthritis* for the word *asthma* in the foregoing paragraphs, this will to a great extent reflect the current state of affairs in the traditional, drug-oriented management of arthritis.

In the case of skin allergies, local warmth and flushing may be caused when the circular muscles in the walls of the arteries that bring the blood to the area are relaxed (dilated), and allowing an increased flow of warm blood into the tissues supplied by the dilated arteries. The skin is pale, becomes cold, and may even get numb and blue when the circular muscles contract and the vessels are constricted, reducing the local blood supply. Reynaud's disease is a form of allergic arterial blood vessel spasm that restricts the flow of blood to the limbs and changes in their temperature and color.

Another primary allergic response is overactivity of the mucus-secreting glands in the allergically reacting areas of the body. Increased nasal, postnasal, and eye mucus are noted in cases of allergic sinusitis, chronic rhinitis, and hay fever. At times there is so much thick, drying, sticky bronchial mucus secreted during an attack of asthma that this obstructing substance has to be thinned out by medication, intravenous fluids, steam inhalation, and even bronchial irrigation. There are life-threatening instances when the mucus-filled air passages are almost completely blocked and the bronchial tubes have to be irrigated and suctioned as an emergency measure. The large intestines may produce a lot of mucus during a flare-up of colitis or ileitis, and there may be a considerable amount of mucus, at times blood-tinged or grossly bloody, present in the bowel movement. There are other types of complex immunologic reactions that need not be discussed in this book.

Wherever an allergic reaction occurs in the body, some or all of the symptoms just described may occur. The site of the allergic congestion, muscle spasm, or increased secretion determines the kind of symptoms that will occur. When the offending substances reach the brain, the reaction might be headache, anger, depression, irritability, restlessness, anxiety, dizziness, confusion, fatigue, or disorientation. Those allergens affecting the digestive tract may cause ulcer symptoms, gall-bladder attack, vomiting, indigestion, bloating, cramps, gas, rectal pain or itching, diarrhea, or constipation. Muscles may respond to allergens with soreness, flulike aching, or spasms. And so forth . . . you needn't be prone to the usual allergies like sniffles, sneezing, itching, and rashes to be a seriously affected individual because, as you can see, many kinds of systemic allergic reactions are hidden far within the body and affect many important internal structures.

A very common misconception about allergic reactions to foods is that they are *acute* responses that occur while the offending food is being eaten—or within an hour or so—and some physicians and lay people believe that food allergies are, therefore, not very common and easy to diagnose. This is only a small part of the big picture;

acute, easy-to-diagnose reactions comprise just the tip of the complex food allergy iceberg.

The late Dr. Herbert Rinkel observed several distinct types of food allergies—cyclic, addictive, and fixed. People suffering from what he identified as *cyclic food allergies* can be exposed to a particular dietary allergen or group of them occasionally and not react to the foods even though they are capable of causing important symptoms. If exposure to the same foods continues for as little as three to five days in succession, or if the potential food offenders are eaten two or three times a week, the allergically active factors in the offending foods will accumulate in the system, causing "overload" allergic reactions, and the food-related illness will appear. Arthritis-causing factors that are eaten too often for a particular individual's tolerance will build up to a "critical" level that surpasses the body's threshold of tolerance, and the arthritic individual will experience a local or generalized reaction in the joints, surrounding structures, and muscles. *Potential food allergens can be "activated" by increased frequency of ingestion that causes allergic overloading*.

For example, you may be allergic to potatoes, and yet it is very possible that once every five to seven days, you will be able to eat a large portion of potatoes during a single meal with no ill effects. But if you should eat them every day for a week, it is more than likely that you will come down with some allergic disorders—flulike generalized aches and pains, joint pains, itching, abdominal distention with cramps or nausea, and severe fatigue with headache and depression or general irritability. Or you might dislike store-bought tomatoes and rarely eat them, but when you produce a bumper crop in your garden, you really overdo it and load up for five successive days, then suddenly find yourself flat on your back, feeling restless, nervous, and confused, with a severe migraine headache, a very stuffy nose, ringing in your ears, and nagging muscle and joint pains, and you are just too sick and dizzy to do anything but try to get to the bathroom in time to prevent an "accident" with your loose bowels and/or attacks of urinary urgency.

In cyclic allergies, the symptom-evoking reactions will subside as soon as the internal level of the offending substance drops to a point below the affected person's individual "critical" level—his or her allergic threshold. As the growing season ends, the excessive ingestion resulting in tomato overexposure ends. And with the passage of time—three or four weeks to several months—a time factor that varies from food to food and is unpredictable in each instance—you may once again tolerate small or even large amounts of the food allergen (tomato) if your food-sensitive (intolerant) tissues are not exposed to this food too frequently thereafter. But if you are not careful, you can easily lose your tolerance again. In most cases the symptoms of cyclic food allergy can be prevented by controlling the interval between exposures. You usually do not have to eliminate the known dietary troublemaker permanently—only long enough to regain a state of tolerance that can be maintained with little difficulty.

Before I was aware of cyclic food allergy and some other aspects of food allergy, I viewed food allergy from what I call the obstetrician's perspective. This is a very simple concept and, for an obstetrician, it is absolutely foolproof. The lady is or is not pregnant—there is no such condition as "just a little pregnant." Herbert Rinkel's discovery of cyclic food allergy taught all of us in clinical ecology that a person might be cyclically allergic to a specific food or group of foods, and at different times might or might *not* have an allergic reaction to a cyclic food allergen. Once it is established, the allergic sensitivity to a particular food is, fortunately, not permanent—"fixed"—in up to eighty percent of the individuals who have food allergy.

The conventional allergist who has the "OB perspective" and is working with a case of food intolerance will, as I used to do, advise the patient to eliminate the offending foods that have clearly been shown in reproducible cause-and-effect observations to have an impact on that individual's physical and mental health.

Over a period of time a food-sensitive person may have compiled an impressive and increasingly restrictive list of foods that he or she is convinced must be avoided in order to remain comfortable. Many nutritious foods are often permanently eliminated from that food-allergic person's diet because they caused important symptoms in the recent or distant past, and there was no awareness of the nature of cyclic food allergy.

The long list of prohibited foods often leads to important long-term problems in diet planning, as the food-intolerant individual, unaware of the positive side of cyclic food allergy, unnecessarily limits the number of foods he or she feels able to eat. In time the "permanent" restriction of many foods leads to *cumulative* allergic food reactions from avoidable and harmful overexposure to previously tolerated foods—the undesirable and preventable effect of the allergic victim's overexposure to a limited selection of formerly "safe" foods. *Food allergy, poorly understood, begets food allergy!*

And things keep getting worse if one is not aware of the plus side of cyclic allergy. In cyclic food allergy there is at least a fifty-fifty chance that tolerance will be regained if the offending foods are avoided for a biologic rest of three weeks to six months. It is not unusual to find that even many of the very worst dietary offenders can be eaten without any ill effects—including the return of your arthritis—if they are not eaten too often. When tolerance to specific foods has been regained, it can be permanent if the former culprits are eaten once every five to seven days. The negative side of reversible cyclic allergy will soon make its unwanted and distressing reappearance—food intolerance—if once again a cumulative (buildup) reaction is deliberately provoked by "overdoing it." In this situation the control of your state of health is really in your *own* hands. In many instances it's entirely up to you whether you have arthritis or not.

This is not a new concept by any means. Twenty-five centuries ago Hippocrates noted "the commencement of a serious disease when they have merely taken twice in the same day the same food which they have been in the custom of taking once." Hippocrates also observed that the ancient Greeks were not harmed by fasting, but after eating certain foods following a fast, they became acutely ill. This observation by the Father of Medicine was accidentally rediscovered by Dr. Rinkel as described in my book, *Dr. Mandell's Five-Day Allergy Relief System*. Dr. Rinkel developed a very useful and accurate diagnostic test for food allergies, the deliberate feeding test, which will be discussed in Chapter 7.

Another type of food allergy is very much like addiction to narcotic drugs. With *addictive food allergies,* unlike the other types of allergies, an allergically addicted person's body actually "needs" and often craves the substance to which it is addictively allergic in order to block or mask the symptoms of addictive withdrawal reactions and maintain a state of comfortable equilibrium. Most people are totally unaware of their addiction-based food dependency. They do not associate the discomfort they experience when deprived of the addicting food allergen with the frequent and very uncomfortable physical and mental symptoms of food withdrawal that accompany this often-encountered addictive disorder.

A woman who is in the habit of eating her favorite food— potatoes—daily may reluctantly eliminate this food when she begins a reducing diet. After a few days she may lose three to ten pounds of allergically retained "water," but she may start to feel ill in a number of ways and experience an almost desperate craving for potatoes. She believes the craving to be evidence of her weak willpower.

She is actually experiencing an addictive withdrawal reaction from a component in the potato that her body's unique chemistry has become dependent upon. Such allergic-addictive cravings may appear several hours or several days after the last meal that contained the addicting food. In addition to her craving for the addicting food, potatoes—a specific symptom—she may also have general withdrawal symptoms like restlessness, irritability, headache, and fatigue.

If she sticks to her diet and fights off the addictive craving for potatoes a few more days and temporarily learns to live with the other uncomfortable symptoms (similar to the "cold turkey" reaction that narcotics addicts experience), her body will recover from the addictive state and no longer demand the relief that could have been experienced if she had ingested potatoes. If she once again begins to eat potatoes too often, she will become "hooked" again. If she should become addicted again, the process will endlessly repeat itself—eating the addicting potato will control her urgent addictive need and produce a temporary feeling of well-being, which will wear off during the withdrawal period and perpetuate the cycle in which she repeatedly requires potatoes again and again for relief of her recurring series of withdrawal reactions caused by her uncontrolled and unsuspected disorder—food addiction.

Many people are aware of their food cravings, and some even shyly or proudly proclaim themselves to be foodoholics, cakeoholics, or chocoholics. They do not recognize their irresistible cravings as characteristic symptoms of addictive food allergy. You may know that you "need" a few slices of bread to clear your head or rid yourself of a daily morning headache, but you do not realize that the wheat or yeast in the much-needed bread is an addicting food—an important allergen that causes the delayed appearance of withdrawal symptoms to occur in your brain with monotonous regularity every morning. Compulsive drinkers (alcoholics) or chain smokers are often well aware of their addictions without realizing that allergies lie at the base of them. The same applies to millions of allergic arthritics, who notice that their pain and stiffness will always worsen (acute reaction) or improve (masking of symptoms) after they have eaten a certain food, taken a particular beverage, or stayed in a specific "chemically polluted" environment.

The third type of allergy pinpointed by Dr. Rinkel is the one with which lay people are most familiar: the *fixed allergy*. Every time you eat a particular food, such as milk, strawberries, or pork, or inhale certain pollens and molds, or absorb an active chemical substance such as paint fumes, hair spray, perfume, gasoline, or exterminating fluid, you have a predictable reaction in certain body systems. What the lay persons may not know, however, is the extremely wide range of symptoms that such reactions can encompass. As you can see from the questionnaire beginning on page 95, allergic reactions extend far beyond the sniffles, sneezes, itching, and rash category to include the allergic reactions in arthritic joints and nearby body structures.

Pages 233–234 list some of the most common food allergens to which many people may be sensitive individually or in combination; page 187 lists common environmental offenders. When you combine the information on the list of allergens with the vast array of possible reactions they can provoke, you can understand why clinical ecologists maintain that many of the physical and mental disorders suffered by millions of people today are allergic in nature. After all, it certainly makes sense, doesn't it? Once humans lived in an environment containing little but the same natural substances of which their bodies were made, so there was very little foreign chemical matter against which the body had to defend itself with an allergic reaction. Nutrition was limited to what the growing season and simple storage systems could provide, so diets of fresh foods were, in a sense, automatically rotated, and this prevented the appearance of numerous cumulative allergic reactions.

Today, however, thanks to modern technology, year-round exposure is possible because of contemporary transportation and storage methods. We can eat the foods to which we are addicted or sensitive, and along with them, we consume a dizzying array of artificial, laboratory-produced chemicals that color them, flavor them, preserve them, "enhance" them, or actually create them. Also, almost every day a new product or by-product of man's brilliant chemical technology is added to the increasingly polluted twentieth-century environment in which we exist: petroleum-based polyester fabrics instead of cotton; auto exhausts instead of horse aromas; plastics instead of wood, stone, or glass.

If the human body could evolve and adapt as quickly as technology invents, many of us would be able to tolerate rather than have to fight off the effects of these and myriad other products of scientific "advances" that fill our environment. But the process of evolution is slow in adjusting to environmental offenders, so the individual body must defend itself against whatever it cannot tolerate—and it often does so via an "allergic" response.

How do we determine what, if any, allergies a person has? Since the early days of allergic medicine, solutions—allergenic extracts—

have been prepared from animal dander and the hair of horses, cattle, hogs, goats, cats, and stray dogs; other extracts are prepared from various molds and the pollens of many species of trees, grasses, and weeds. During testing for allergies, small amounts of these solutions or extracts were scratched or injected into the outer layer of a patient's skin. If a hivelike wheal or an area of redness developed at the test site, an allergy to the particular animal, mold, or pollen source of the extract was suspected.

The skin reaction at the test area is currently interpreted as objective evidence that the body's misinformed immune system has produced unnecessary specific allergic antibodies to fight off the nonthreatening natural airborne substances. It has incorrectly "recognized" the testing extracts as carriers of the biologically active, supposedly harmful offenders that it tried to dispose of before they caused any adverse effects. Allergic reactions to harmless environmental substances may be viewed as evidence of an overactive immunologic defense mechanism; but it's not quite that simple, and there are exceptions. Most allergy patients were advised to dispose of pets, stay away from animals, move away or stay indoors during the pollen seasons, take desensitizing allergy shots, or simply to live with it with the help of various medications. Skin tests, however, are not as accurate as we allergists would like them to be (food skin tests are generally regarded to be only 20% accurate—an error of 80%!) and they cannot show us which particular symptoms are caused by specific allergic reactions to different offenders.

Many patients who have been told they had no allergies because of negative conventional skin tests, especially for foods and molds, have been shown to be highly sensitive to these allergens when tested by the symptom-duplicating provocative-testing methods employed by clinical ecologists. A widely respected pioneer in ecologic medicine, my distinguished friend and teacher Dr. Carleton Lee, discovered the symptom-relieving/neutralizing technique that often eliminated the symptoms of active allergies within a few minutes. This was a giant step in the diagnosis of internal allergies, because now we could often stop or reduce the intensity of reactions brought on by provocative testing or a presenting illness. On occasion, using Lee's neutralization technique, I have been able to clear a new patient's symptoms—temporarily—on the first visit. Dr. Lee's system was useful, but the intradermal injections in the outer layer of the skin were a little uncomfortable for some of the patients, especially young children. At times some skin tests with highly colored food extracts would leave a small area of food pigment at the test site. The use of sublingual tests eliminated these problems. The thin-walled sublingual veins on the floor of the mouth just under the top of the tongue in the area behind the lower front teeth are very absorbent and close to the surface. Ecologists Dr. Guy O. Pfeiffer and Dr. Lawrence D. Dickey adopted the needle-free technique of Dr. French Hansel, in which small amounts of carefully measured drops of allergenic extracts are placed under the tongue. Just as a thermometer placed under the tongue accurately and without discomfort registers internal temperature quickly, sublingual tests will often duplicate with great accuracy the various symptoms caused by a patient's allergies. The test materials consist of drops of extracts prepared from frequently eaten foods, common airborne molds, pollens, and the like, and solutions prepared from environmental chemicals that are often encountered in daily living.

Provocative nasal inhalation tests are a very sensitive diagnostic measure that Dr. Harris Hosen suggested I become familiar with in 1956. During testing dry, powdered airborne allergens like house dust; animal dander; tree, grass and weed pollens; and various molds are sniffed deeply into the patient's nose. They travel up the tear ducts to the surface of the eyes and to the depths of the bronchial tubes. They often cause diagnostically valuable local symptoms when they contact the allergically sensitive cells in the eyes and respiratory tract. They also induce important symptoms throughout the body after they are absorbed into the circulation from the upper respiratory tract and the intestines.

Since the beginnings of the practice of allergy medicine, the production of allergenic extracts and the preparation of other test materials have been developed to the point that we are now able to test a patient safely for over three hundred sensitivities from apple to banana to auto exhaust, tobacco smoke, and yellow food coloring as well as pollens, dust, dander, and so on.

Whatever symptom-duplicating diagnostic-testing technique is used by the ecologist (intradermal, sublingual, inhalation, or deliberate-feeding challenges), the general principle is one of producing a patient's familiar symptoms by "provocation" with unidentified (to the patient) testing solutions to demonstrate a clear-cut cause-and-effect relationship with the single-blind technique. Provocative challenges with substances the patient has known responses to that result in the prompt appearance of familiar manifestations of that patient's illness provide very convincing clinical evidence of the etiology or cause(s) of the disorder. This evidence is corroborated by the success of treatment that is directed against the substances that were identified during provocative testing as the probable cause of particular symptoms.

With our cause-and-effect diagnostic approach, we have demonstrated this evidence to be scientifically valid in our successful conservative, drug-free management program, which is directed at the specific underlying causes of each individual's illness due to widespread but generally unsuspected allergy. Once we have determined a profile of the substances to which a given person is sensitive, and we have established what symptoms each of these substances is causing, we devise an overall plan to remove the offenders from his or her body and environment or minimize their effects if they cannot be avoided or eliminated. In addition to prescribing patient-specific diets and environmental modifications, we give desensitizing allergy treatments (shots or immunotherapy) and increase "allergic resistance" by a number of methods, including general supportive and allergy-oriented nutritional therapy.

Are allergic symptoms relieved by eliminating certain foods and beverages or making changes in the patient's environment? If so, that gives us additional important information to work with. One by one, we fully investigate all the diagnostic clues obtained from medical histories during consultation and confirm our provocative-test results as we introduce the test-identified probable offenders again into the patient's system, either by retesting sublingually or by observing what happens after returning or adding foods to the diet or chemicals to the environment.

Whatever substance causes allergic or allergylike reactions is considered, with very little doubt (there is always some doubt in science), to be an offending environmental factor related to the physical and/or mental disorder at hand. And with the assistance of my technicians and nurses, I help the patient formulate a comprehensive treatment program and way of life that eliminates or minimizes the effect of the offenders, with a high degree of success in the majority of cooperating patients.

In offices, clinics, and hospital environmental units around the country, more and more doctors are using these simple and accurate ecological techniques to diagnose and treat a wide variety of allergylike, previously unexplainable physical and mental ailments, including presumed "psychosomatic" disorders as well as thousands of cases of arthritis.

5

How Allergies Cause Arthritis

"Arthritis an allergy? That's crazy!" "It's impossible." "I never heard that one before." These are common reactions among both lay people and health professionals, at least until they've seen and understood the easily demonstrated connection between arthritis and allergy. Clinical ecologists have shown that in 80 to 90 percent of arthritis cases, allergy is the culprit. It has been scientifically proved by the recently published double-blind study I conducted with the assistance of Anthony Conte, M.D., which confirms my previous observations and those of other ecologists.*

The mechanism is the same as for any other allergic reaction. Remember that the pain, swelling, and stiffness in arthritic joints (and ultimately the permanent damage) are due to an excess of fluid in and around the joints and the joint inflammation that occurs when the body attempts to defend itself against the environmental offender. When a substance to which the body is sensitive arrives at an affected or soon-to-be-affected joint via the bloodstream, the capillaries in the synovial membrane lining the joint (see diagram of a typical joint on page 42) respond with an inflammatory reaction,

*Marshall Mandell, M.D., and Anthony Conte, M.D., "The Role of Allergy in Arthritis, Rheumatism, and Polysymptomatic Cerebral, Visceral and Somatic Disorders: A Double-Blind Study," *Journal of the International Academy of Preventative Medicine* (July 1982).

allowing fluid and certain cells from the bloodstream to enter the joint and the surrounding tissues. This occurs because the immune system begins an unnecessary, illness-causing effort to fight off the usually harmless substance it unfortunately recognizes as an offending intruder.

I first became aware of the allergy-arthritis connection in my own practice about twenty years ago.* The connection was observed during the course of testing a sixty-one-year-old woman to determine the causes of her allergic bronchial asthma. She was undergoing a series of provocative sublingual tests during which I expected to evoke asthmatic symptoms that would identify the substances responsible for the frequent and distressing attacks of this lower respiratory tract allergy.

Within a few minutes after administering the first dose of corn extract to see if this very common cereal grain might be a factor in her asthmatic condition, I was quite surprised when, instead of provoking an episode of asthma, the test caused an episode of joint pain and stiffness in her left ankle. When I asked her if she had ever had any problems of this type in her left ankle previously, she certainly was not puzzled about the matter. Firmly but politely she replied, "Young man, that is my arthritis!"

Several experiences of this nature quickly taught me that I should take more complete histories of my allergic patients in order to anticipate the very likely appearance of test-provoked symptoms of other familiar ailments—not the presenting symptoms that brought them to me—that conventional, mainstream medicine had never even suspected might be of allergic origin. Soon after I began to perform those remarkably illuminating symptom-duplicating tests—and repeated them to prove that they were reproducible—I realized how common internal and cerebral allergies were. I had an exciting opportunity to provoke and study firsthand numerous predictable episodes of physical and mental disorders in my own office—on schedule. I was amazed to learn how many important ailments actually were unrecognized allergies. The underlying allergic-ecologic causes of many forms of serious illness had been completely overlooked by the entire medical profession, with few excep-

*Describing this first case of allergic-ecologic arthritis in my practice does not imply that I discovered the allergy-arthritis connection. I "rediscovered" for myself what others had already observed, and what was reported almost twenty years previously by Dr. Michael Zeller. The subject has been studied extensively and augmented by my mentor, the pioneering Dr. Theron G. Randolph, who was associated with Dr. Zeller and Dr. Rinkel for many years.

tions. And it was now obvious that physicians covering up symptoms with drugs were not treating these disorders correctly, since they had no idea of the underlying factors that had to be managed in order to control the illness. I confirmed this extremely important relationship between environmental factors and many disorders of body and mind an impressive number of times as I tested and retested my patients.

In many cases it will be easy for an arthritic person such as yourself to determine if his or her arthritis is an allergic disorder. And once it has been shown to your satisfaction that this is the case, it is usually not very difficult to relieve your pain and swelling. In addition, you will probably be able to prevent the occurrence of permanent joint damage, or at least keep it limited in severity as you bring the allergies under control by yourself or with professional assistance.

Thousands of cases of allergic arthritis have been diagnosed by clinical ecologists in the United States, Canada, England, Australia, and elsewhere. Allergic arthritis is a common disorder, and it may very well be the kind that you have. When you become familiar with the contents of the next section of this book, you will have the information that is needed to set up and carry out your own arthritis self-help program of diagnosis and treatment.

It is very likely that many of my readers will be able to do everything in the Lifetime Arthritis System from start to finish on their own and be well again, or much better, without any professional assistance. If your self-help program is not completely successful, at least there is an excellent chance that you will learn so much about your illness, even if it happens to be a very complex disorder, that you will strongly suspect or have definitely proved that you are allergic and are proceeding in the right direction, even though it is obvious that additional help is necessary. After reading this book you will know a great deal about arthritis, what to do and where to go to obtain the relief you seek—the greatest relief possible without drugs, surgery, or radiation.

Do not settle for partial relief of your arthritis if a slight to moderate improvement is the "final" result of your self-help program. Of course, it will be good to see the swollen joints reduced in size. And it certainly will be wonderful to have less pain and be able to move about more freely, with better use of your hands and limbs. And it will be great to be able to bend your neck and back more than you could only one week before.

These welcome changes, which you may be able to bring about

through your own efforts, will be an exciting breakthrough in the course of your arthritis. Together we will have proved that your illness, with its associated misery, is at the very least partially reversible. We will have accomplished a bit of medical magic in a few days: we will have brought into being a partial remission that nobody can call spontaneous because we planned this happy event in advance. After years of illness, your arthritis will really improve—and *you* will have done it.

You, your loved ones, and your friends will be pleased, perhaps overjoyed, by your improvement. So will I. But I will not let you stop there, for there is no reason to be satisfied that a moderate improvement is the best that can be accomplished.

Let's go for the brass ring—complete or near-complete, natural (drug-free, if possible) control over your arthritis. Let's make a major effort to *cure* this painful number-one crippler. It's going to take time, effort, and money, but the odds are greatly in your favor, and considering what might be accomplished, it certainly is worth trying. Haven't we already established that your arthritis, and perhaps some other important ailments and/or symptoms, are reversible, allergic-ecologic disorders?

The next step is to get professional help from an experienced ecologist. Some cases of arthritis and some cases of nonarthritic ecologic diseases (affecting other parts and systems of the body) are so complicated that they positively require the expertise of a well-trained, ecologically oriented physician. A regular allergist—even a board-certified specialist such as I was in my preecology days—does not have the knowledge and skill to help you. In fact, there's a very good chance that if you were to discuss an ecologic evaluation with a conventional, traditional allergist, the allergist would probably try to discourage you with negative comments the same way the conventional internists and rheumatologists tried to discourage Dr. Ford from going to Dr. Randolph's unit, where he achieved such wonderful results. And don't be surprised if he or she becomes upset when you say that you have an appointment to consult with a clinical ecologist about your allergic arthritis and that you are going to be tested comprehensively to identify all the dietary and environmental substances which you are often exposed to that could be responsible for your allergic-ecologic arthritis.

Traditionally trained allergists have never been exposed to, or have not taken the opportunity to become familiar with, the currently available information concerning the often easy to demonstrate causes of environmentally produced arthritis. Few medical schools teach anything at all about ecologic science (the clinical application of ecologic principles), and there is not very much instruction about allergy, preventive medicine, or clinical nutrition given to our future doctors.

It is understandable how many fine, sincere physicians are not nearly as effective as they could be despite their intellectual capacity and desire to help their patients. Their diagnostic and therapeutic horizons are greatly limited by these generally unrecognized deficiencies in their training.

The Arthritis Foundation, which is a major source of information for interested physicians and the public, has flatly rejected the idea that arthritis could be an allergic disorder of the joints and muscles. The foundation does not or will not believe that arthritis might be associated with, or caused by reactions to or a lack of, certain substances in the diet. I have previously mentioned that the foundation does believe that an allergylike immunologic reaction caused by factors unknown to them may be responsible for arthritis, but they continue to ignore the dietary and environmental factors that ecologists have clearly shown in thousands of instances are capable of setting off attacks of arthritis. This is a very puzzling inconsistency.

Be that as it may, you can judge the facts for yourself and make up your own mind.

I wish to emphasize the fact that every disease must have a cause. A good way of determining that our testing for the causes of arthritis by provocative techniques is accurate and clinically effective is to see if application of this information leads to a treatment that cures or significantly relieves an active case or prevents its recurrence. That is exactly what clinical ecologists have done for many years in case after case and study after study with thousands of patients. We do not claim to be able to cure the bone damage associated with arthritis if the allergy-initiated inflammation and structural changes are allowed to continue too long, but we can give considerable relief to many. Together, the arthritic and the ecologist often cure arthritis by continuous attention to the demonstrable causes in each case, while the condition remains in its reversible state. Careful avoidance of test-identified food offenders in conjunction with a rotary-diversified diet, desensitization treatment (immunotherapy), and changes in life-style, along with nutritional supplements, can prevent the occurrence of future "spontaneous" flare-ups due to exposure to previously unsuspected dietary and environmental factors.

For four decades clinical ecologists have been diagnosing and successfully treating allergic and allergylike arthritis by determining the specific foods and the other environmental factors that caused or exacerbated the disease in each individual case.

Drs. Theron G. Randolph (who practices in Chicago) and Michael Zeller (who practiced in Chicago until his death in 1978) pioneered this work in the 1940s. After testing a large group of rheumatoid and osteoarthritic sufferers for food sensitivities, they relieved many of their symptoms by eliminating the arthritis-inducing factors from the diet and then observed the *recurrence* of those symptoms when the offending foods were reintroduced. There was nothing "spontaneous" here; it was a clearly demonstrated cause-and-effect situation. Since then Dr. Randolph has significantly improved 80 to 90 percent of a group of about a thousand patients having rheumatoid arthritis. He found food allergy to be the major factor in many of these cases. He also discovered that allergylike sensitivity to many common chemical substances was a very important although previously unrecognized factor in the causation of arthritis and many other kinds of illness. This discovery was a major contribution to the practice of medicine and goes far beyond arthritis in its clinical application. Working together, Dr. Randolph and Dr. Kendall Gerdes, who practices in Denver, found that food allergy and chemical susceptibility were also involved in cases of osteoarthritis.

In another joint effort, Drs. Randolph and Gerdes recently completed a follow-up study of several hundred arthritis patients whom they had treated ten years previously. Sixty-eight percent of the patients reported a continued long-term improvement of 75 to 100 percent compared with their pretreatment condition; 15 percent said their arthritis had improved from 50 percent to 74 percent. Only 8 patients said their condition had not improved.

Other similarly oriented doctors have demonstrated that not only are the benefits of the ecologic approach to arthritis effective over the long term, but they work for a broad cross-section of the population. During his forty-plus years of practice, for instance, Dr. Carleton Lee of St. Joseph, Missouri, an early researcher in clinical ecology who discovered the technique of neutralizing symptoms by administering small doses of the substance that caused them, relieved or eliminated arthritis symptoms from over six thousand allergic patients.

Controlled laboratory experiments have confirmed the connection between allergy and arthritis. In my own arthritis research project with Dr. Anthony Conte, we employed the scientifically accepted method of double-blind testing to confirm objectively my twenty years of clinical observations that acute episodes of painful arthritis symptoms (joint and muscle pain, stiffness, swelling, and limited motion of joints and fatigue) can be provoked by the sublingual administration of allergenic extracts, and solutions of various chemical substances. In performing these simple arthritis-inducing challenges, neither the arthritic people being tested nor the technicians administering the symptom-duplicating tests knew what substances were being used.

In some instances drops of food and inhalant extracts (dust, molds, pollens) or chemical solutions that might be causes of the arthritic patients' condition were placed under the tongue. In other tests, for purposes of scientific control, a placebo of sterile triple distilled water was given. In 87.5 percent of the arthritic volunteers tested, familiar arthritis symptoms were duplicated by this controlled exposure to common substances to which the patient might well be exposed on a daily basis. Placebos in almost every case caused no reactions.

At the Southeastern Chronic Disease Center in Chadbourn, North Carolina, Drs. Murray Carroll and Thurman Bullock carefully studied the role of foods and chemicals in over three hundred individuals suffering from rheumatoid arthritis and osteoarthritis in the environmentally controlled section of their hospital. These clinical researchers found that in 98 percent of the osteo patients and 91 percent of the RA (rheumatoid) patients, arthritis symptoms improved materially in the controlled hospital environment when the specific foods that these arthritic individuals were allergic to were removed from their diets. And their arthritis symptoms were acutely exacerbated, along with the symptoms of other, previously unrecognized and misdiagnosed chronic or recurrent internal allergic disorders—headache, fatigue, nervousness, depression, and disorders of the respiratory and digestive tracts—when these patients with severe food allergy were given a series of single-food deliberate-feeding challenges.

These arthritic patients had acute reactions after ingesting the foods to which they were allergic after these specific foods had been removed from their diets for five days or longer. This technique of single-food testing after eliminating the offending foods (the deliberate feeding test, or DFT) converts chronic symptoms into diagnostically significant acute flare-ups that are usually characterized by many signs and symptoms. Among the most important reactions in this study were the objective physical changes in the involved arthritic joints and muscles, which were identical with the patients' familiar arthritic manifestations. The deliberate feeding test is an invaluable diagnostic measure that is frequently used by clinical ecologists; it was developed by our trailblazing clinical researcher, Herbert Rinkel, M.D.

In 1980 Drs. Carroll and Bullock, in a joint project with two other groups of prominent clinical ecologists, Dr. George Kroker and Dr. Theron G. Randolph, and Dr. William Rea and his associates tested three separate groups of rheumatoid arthritis patients in their environmentally controlled, hospital-based ecologic units located in North Carolina, Illinois, and Texas. After each patient's symptoms were relieved or eliminated by therapeutic fasting on spring water in the unpolluted atmosphere of the ecology units, each group of investigators was able to induce self-limited episodes of familiar arthritic symptoms in all the subjects. This was accomplished by administering single-food deliberate-feeding challenges or by exposing the arthritic patients to various chemical agents. Changes in joint size, muscle strength, intensity of pain, and laboratory findings, such as eosinophile counts, sedimentation tests, RA factors, and Reactive Protein, conducted before and after test meals and chemical exposures, were carefully documented.

In their reports to the American Rheumatism Association and the American College of Allergists, Dr. Randolph and Dr. Rea hypothesized that the underlying cause of arthritis related to foods and environmental chemicals was the "increased permeability of various membranes" due to allergic sensitivity to environmental factors.

Outside the field of clinical ecology, the same connection between allergy and arthritis was made by a very observant clinician, Dr. I-Tsu Chao, a fellow of the American Academy of Allergy who practices in New York City. In 1981 he presented an excellent paper to the American College of Allergists in which he reported his independent research findings that "commonly consumed foods" were a major cause of chronic arthritis. In 1959, about five years before I provoked my first episode of allergic arthritis with corn extract, Dr. I-Tsu Chao discovered the connection accidentally. He noticed that the arthritic symptoms of many patients with this condition were relieved by the special diets that he designed to control the manifestations of the other forms of food allergy that they were being treated for. Since then he has performed a carefully controlled double-blind investigation on arthritic patients and found that "remissions and exacerbations of arthritis and other associated symptoms could be induced at will by dietary manipulation."

In other words, these previously misunderstood variations in the course of chronic arthritis are not what the Arthritis Foundation and mainstream medicine persist in mislabeling as spontaneous remissions and unexplained flare-ups. The remissions are predictable improvements that can be turned on and off by eliminating the specific dietary allergens responsible for the illness. All these cases and studies clearly show that in an overwhelming majority of arthritic patients, the cause of arthritis is not unknown. In most instances the cause(s) of this crippling disease—affecting almost 400,000,000 people—can be accurately identified in one to two weeks by a competent clinical ecologist.

Not all "traditional" rheumatologists are rigidly opposed to new approaches; they keep their minds open to new developments. But it helps drive the point home when they find out for themselves. Dr. Franklin C. Anderson, for instance, is a midwestern physician who was nearly crippled with rheumatoid arthritis that seriously interfered with the performance of his practice. It was hard for him to get around, and his hands were so badly affected that he was unable to perform examinations. His case resisted all treatment, including the methods employed by the world-renowned Mayo Clinic. By chance Dr. Anderson learned of Dr. Theron G. Randolph, and he entered the ecologic unit in Illinois. As soon as the offending foods were eliminated from his system by a few days of fasting on pure spring water in the controlled environment, he reports, "Results were dramatic. I could hardly believe them." He could move his hands, and stand and sit easily for the first time in years. In an open letter to patients and fellow arthritics, Dr. Anderson wrote, "My symptoms were turned on and off like a switch. Unbelievable!" He did believe it because it was a demonstrable fact—he got well. With the knowledge he gained from his ecologic studies under Dr. Randolph's and Dr. Kroker's care, he is happy and comfortable. He is once again working at his practice full-time and enjoying the greatly enhanced quality of his life.

Dr. Anderson controls his arthritis by giving very careful attention to the rotary diversified diet by which he regulates the interval between his exposure to each food that could cause his arthritis to flare up if it were to be eaten too often and build up in his body to a level greater than that which his allergic joints and muscles can tolerate. It is very likely that you, too, can discover that there is a clear-cut cause-and-effect relationship between a currently active state of food allergy and/or chemical sensitivity and your arthritis.

First, do you have arthritis? Have you been diagnosed as arthritic? Do you have any of the most common symptoms of arthritis? Pain and stiffness in one or more joints, especially on arising?

Persistent swelling and tenderness and limited motion in one or more joints? Pain and stiffness in a joint that was once injured? Do these symptoms come and go, apparently with no reason? Do you experience unexplainable fatigue or a low-grade fever that also comes and goes?

One or a combination of those symptoms is a good indicator of arthritis in one of its many forms. As I have already explained, it is important to treat those symptoms *early,* before permanent joint damage can develop.

Do you, or did you, have any allergies, past or present, like eczema, hay fever, asthma, or hives? Or do any close relatives have a history of allergies? Do you have frequent "indigestion" or nasal and sinus congestion? Do you seem to suffer colds or flu more often than others? Do you have other health problems, like migraine headaches, colitis, unexplained fatigue or bodywide complaints, or other chronic symptoms that may be undiagnosed allergies?

If your answer to any of these questions is yes, then it is possible that your arthritis is allergic in origin, but you must understand that allergic arthritis may occur in the absence of these conditions. By carefully and thoroughly following the instructions in the next section of this book, it is likely that you will be able to pinpoint the substances causing your arthritis if, as is true in 80 to 90 percent of arthritis cases, it falls in the category of being caused by allergy or allergylike sensitivity or intolerance to foods or chemical and/or airborne substances.

If you can identify the major causes of your condition among these substances, there is an excellent chance that you will find relief from your arthritis. Even if you are not able to discover *all* the dietary and environmental causes of your allergic-ecologic arthritis, you may identify enough of them to reduce significantly the "total load" on your body. Your joints and muscles may be considerably better as the allergic stress is decreased by elimination, reduction, or control of important offending substances.

Section II

How to Relieve Allergic Arthritis

Before You Begin . . .

The bioecologic approach to arthritis control is the safest available approach because it does not add drugs that Professor A. H. Corwin, Professor emeritus of chemistry at Johns Hopkins University, classes as "selective poisons" to the body or that make any other physical intrusions. But the self-help system we are going to use to determine which allergens produce your arthritic response may place some stress on some individuals. If you have a serious medical problem other than your arthritis—if you have heart trouble, diabetes, asthma, epilepsy, or a recent history of serious emotional problems such as severe or suicidal depression or violence or self-destructive behavior—you must protect yourself and others by being tested under the supervision of an ecologically trained physician or clinic. You will find a list of such specialists at the back of the book.

At the very least, if you have any serious doubts about the overall state of your health, you should consult with and be examined by your physician before beginning the self-tests.

Remember that many doctors are unaware of the effectiveness of our approach and may try to dissuade you from this course of action even after giving you a clean bill of health.

Also remember that many kinds of nonarthritic symptoms often are themselves unrecognized allergic reactions or allergylike responses, which will disappear along with your arthritis when trigger substances are eliminated.

In any case, use your good common sense. After all, you wouldn't sign up for a vigorous physical fitness program, no matter how good you believe it might make you feel, if you were still recovering from a heart attack or a broken leg! When in doubt, consult your physician.

Besides common sense, you will need to call on your intelligence and your self-awareness. I am going to ask you to be a detective and to look for clues in your own body. You will need to be alert to reactions as you work your way through the Lifetime Arthritis Relief program. When it is appropriate, ask for help from a friend or relative who cares about you and will check on your condition several times each day to see if you need any assistance and to follow your progress and learn about your observations.

If you are like most people, you will be surprised to learn that you probably already *know* the cause of your arthritis! It has been my experience that at least three fourths of the patients who come to my office will bring invaluable diagnostic-clue-laden information with them. Some cases are very easy for me; others can be a little "tricky"; and some are difficult and complex.

Patients often reveal their allergies and their addictions. "I've never been able to tolerate milk." "My knees hurt like the devil about two hours after I eat pork." And one might say, "I love tomatoes so much that I could eat them with every meal." And sure enough, one has a severe reaction to the dairy-products tests, one has "pork arthritis," and the other shows extreme sensitivity to tomatoes. "Food X always relieves my headache." "I start to ache if I skip a meal." "I feel wonderful if I fast." "Two ounces of beer and the pain in my knuckles and elbows disappears." "I can't stand fresh paint, hair spray, and bus fumes."

Your answers to the questionaires in the next chapter will serve as your guide to discovering the cause or at least some of the important causes of your allergic-ecologic arthritis symptoms. After providing yourself with that basic information, you will find instructions in the succeeding chapters for the three stages of your individualized arthritis-relief program:

1. clearing the body of all possible allergens
2. testing for arthritis triggers
3. planning for a lifetime free from arthritis

If at first glance the process seems too complicated or arduous, read it over again and think about it, because it really is easy. Remind yourself that a few weeks of effort are a very small price to pay for many years of good health and freedom from pain and possible crippling. I also wish to reassure you at the outset that in all likelihood you will not have to give up permanently most of those favorite foods and some of the activities that presently cause your arthritis flare-ups. Once the food-allergic arthritic person's body is thoroughly free of the effects of the specific group of offending foods (after a period of food elimination that gives you a much-needed biologic rest from allergy stress), you, like most other food-sensitive patients, will find that you can tolerate many of them in the near future without suffering reactions.

Your comfort and health are now to a great degree in your own hands. One advantage of the bioecologic approach to arthritis and other allergic-ecologic disorders is that it gives you—the one who was always on the scene in the arthritic body (rather than a doctor or a pharmacist)—the full-time, major responsibility for improving your own health and well-being in a conservative, drug-free way. With my help, I know that you can easily assume that responsibility and do an excellent job as you seriously proceed through the system that I devised, as detailed in the next chapters.

6

Finding Clues to Your
Allergy-Related Arthritis

Your answers to the questions in this chapter will help you discover whether you are among the 80 percent of arthritis sufferers who can be helped by my bioecologic system.

You may be surprised by some of the questions and wonder how they relate to your arthritis symptoms. As I've previously explained, it has been the experience of my colleagues and myself that arthritis is often only one among many allergic reactions, so other symptoms in other areas or systems can be indications of overall allergic sensitivity. When you eventually pinpoint and eliminate the dietary and environmental factors that trigger your allergic-ecologic arthritis, you will probably be pleasantly surprised to find that some other seemingly unrelated disorders will disappear, too.

The first step in your arthritis-relief program is to determine if your arthritis symptoms are due to allergic or allergylike reactions, so please think carefully while you are answering the following questions.*

1. Since many childhood allergies change form as one grows

*I have modified the questionnaire in "Chronic Urticaria: The Role of Food Allergy" by Alfred V. Zamm, M.D., published in *Clinical Ecology* (also published in *Cutis* magazine). Reprinted from *Cutis 9 (1972):257; by permission of author and publisher.*

older, it may be that your arthritis flare-ups now are different kinds of sensitivity reactions to substances that used to cause unrecognized allergic health problems when you were young. So think back to your childhood and check with your parents, older brothers and sisters, and so on.

Yes No

Did you have hives?

Did you wet the bed?

Did you have eczema or any other chronic skin trouble?

Did you have colic?

Were you a feeding problem?

Did you have frequent earaches?

Did you have croup?

Did you have frequent bronchitis or chest colds?

Did you have persistent (day or night) coughs?

Did you have hay fever?

Did you have frequent attacks of "stomachache," diarrhea, or vomiting?

Did you have circles under the eyes?

Did you have learning disabilities?

Did you rub your nose from side to side with your finger or with the back of your hand ("saluting")?

Did you have a stuffy nose?

Did you have growing pains?

Were you hyperactive?

Did you have asthma?

Did you have epilepsy?

Did you have facial pallor?

Did you have headaches?

Did you have mood swings?   Yes   No

Did you have bad behavior not under your control?

Did you have reading problems (LD, dyslexia)?

Did you have a short attention span?

Did you have frequent nosebleeds?

A *yes* answer to any of these questions indicates that you may have been allergic as a child and that your present arthritis may be an adult conversion or equivalent of that childhood allergy.

2. Now you will explore your current or recent patterns of possible and probable allergies, of which your arthritis may be a part.

                                                                Yes   No

a. Gastrointestinal system:
Have you frequently belched or passed gas after
   meals?

Have you often had indigestion and bloating or
   abdominal distension after meals?

Is there any food that you feel disagrees with you
   often or each time you eat it?

Have you often had attacks of diarrhea?

Have you often had constipation or chronic constipation?

Have you suffered with cramping pains in your
   abdomen?

Have you ever been told you have spastic or
   mucous colitis? Ileitis? Ulcer?

Have you ever been told you have gall bladder or
   bile duct disease?

Have you ever had acute pain in the abdomen
   associated with headache, fatigue, dizziness,
   depression, hives, or itching of the skin?

b. Food: Yes No

Have you suspected any food of causing or aggravating your condition?

Have you or did you go on eating binges or "food jags"?

Are there any foods that you dislike or hate?

Are there any foods you crave, love, overindulge in, or eat frequently because you like them so much?

Is there any seasonal food (for example, strawberries, corn, tomatoes, peaches, etc.) that you overindulge in?

Are there any foods you find difficult to digest?

Have any foods you eat caused nausea, vomiting, diarrhea, heartburn, belching, gas, cramps, hives, skin rashes, headache?

Are you uncomfortable or ill if you do not eat on time?

Have you a sense of well-being after you eat?

Are you more alert or energetic after eating?

Have you felt better if you skipped a meal or fasted?

Has fasting ever relieved any symptoms?

Are you uncomfortable or sick when you fast?

Have you felt good after a three- to five-day fast?

c. Alcohol:

Do alcoholic beverages take any kind of symptoms away?

Do you get a hangover from a single drink?

Do you need to drink an alcoholic beverage at least once a day to relax or be comfortable?

Do you find you crave an alcoholic beverage?

Do you drink the same type of alcoholic beverage   Yes No
  every time you drink?

Has any drink ever made you ill or caused any kind
  of symptom?

Does any alcoholic beverage make you ill now, or
  when you were first learning to drink?

Do complaints appear a short time after you drink?

Do symptoms appear hours after you drink?

Do symptoms appear the following morning?

Does an alcoholic beverage at any time relieve any
  physical or mental discomfort that you may
  have?

Does even a small amount of alcohol have an effect
  on you?

Does alcohol affect you if it is taken with certain
  foods?

Are you an alcoholic?

Have you had any of the following symptoms?

                                           Yes No

  d. Skin:
  itching?

  flushing?

  pallor?

  rash?

  hives?

  acne?

  tingling/burning sensation?

  eczema?

e. Eyes: Yes   No
itching?

burning?

red/congested?

puffy lids?

visual blurring?

dark circles (shiners)?

tearing?

mucus discharge?

crusted lids?

feeling of "sand" in your eyes?

f. Ear, nose, throat, chest:
popping or ringing in ears?

frequent ear infections?

itching in ears?

excessive ear wax?

fluid in ears?

ears feel blocked/clogged?

Menière's disease?

hearing decreased?

sounds too loud?

nasal discharge?

postnasal drip?

sneezing?

itchy nose?

sinus pressure?

nasal obstruction?

sore throat?

hoarseness?   Yes   No

laryngitis?

coughing?

dryness in throat?

frequent clearing of throat?

sense of smell lost?

sense of smell very acute?

sinuses obstructed/full?

sinus pain?

frequent colds?

chest congestion?

chest pain?

tightness in chest?

shortness of breath?

wheezing?

hay fever?

bronchitis?

frequent pneumonia?

hyperventilation?

asthma?

emphysema?

g. Cardiovascular:
rapid heartbeat?

palpitations?

chest pain?

skipped beats?

hot flashes?

cold extremities?   Yes   No

red, white, or blue hands?

pallor?

flushing?

chills?

h. Genitourinary:
frequent urination?

painful urination?

urgent urination?

lack of bladder control?

bedwetting?

vaginal itching?

vaginal pain?

vaginal discharge?

premenstrual symptoms?

sudden swelling of breasts?

frequent bladder infection?

"nervous bladder"?

kidney disorder(s)?

pain in penis?

pain in testicles?

i. Gastrointestinal:
nausea?

heartburn?

indigestion?

dry mouth?

geographic tongue?

burning or stinging tongue?   Yes   No

burning or stinging mouth?

cold sores/canker sores?

frequent stomach rumbling?

vomiting?

cramps?

diarrhea?

constipation?

ileitis?

colitis?

rectal itching?

rectal burning?

rectal cramps?

frequent burping?

hiccups?

hemorrhoids?

abdominal pain?

bad breath?

bad taste in mouth?

metallic taste?

excessive salivation?

bloating sensation?

visible abdominal distention?

passing excessive gas?

food cravings?

compulsive overeating?

uncontrollable hunger?

uncontrollable thirst?   Yes   No

eating binges?

j. Musculoskeletal:
fatigue?

frequent attacks of "flu" or flu-like illness?

muscle stiffness?

muscle spasm?

muscle soreness?

muscle weakness?

muscle pain?

joint stiffness?

joint swelling?

joint pain?

joint weakness?

backache?

neck ache?

arms heavy?

legs heavy?

pain in arms/legs?

swelling in arms/legs?

redness in arms/legs?

k. Nervous system:
headache?

drowsy or sleepy?

sluggish?

depressed?

anxious?

nervous?   **Yes No**

lack of energy?

restless?

hyperactive?

crying spells?

dizzy?

poor memory?

confusion?

lack of concentration?

poor coordination?

poor comprehension?

angry and/or aggressive behavior?

feeling apart or separate from other people?

feeling that surroundings are unreal?

excessive response to minor emotional stress?

mood swings?

irritable?

unprovoked anger?

seizures?

eyes cross or crossed?

learning disabilities?

eyes track poorly?

short attention span?

clumsy? inept?

poor balance?

mixed dominance (left-handed and right-footed or
 right-handed and left-eyed?)

walked early?

walked late?   Yes   No

talked late?

in playpen most of the time?

in chair/swing most of the time?

on the floor most of the time?

never crawled on floor?

crawled very little before walking?

With the exception of some neurologic findings, a pattern of *yes* answers in any or all sections of this questionnaire is a definite or highly suggestive indication of allergies that affect some part of your body. It is quite likely, but not 100 percent certain, that your joints and associated structures are also being affected by some allergies.

If you came to my office as a patient, we would begin the diagnostic phase of your medical care by having you complete a detailed questionnaire similar to the preceding one. I would review the chronologic history of your health problems since birth, looking for clues and patterns of symptoms. (We ask each patient to prepare this kind of history before his or her first visit.) During our initial consultation I would clarify and enlarge this information by asking a series of detailed questions about the information given in your letters, notes, and questionnaire in order to track down various clues and try to pinpoint the possible environmental and dietary cause of your health problems.

By the end of a forty-five to ninety-minute consultation, with rare exceptions, I have a clear idea of where we will begin our diagnostic testing. By the end of this chapter, you will have a definite indication of where to begin your own testing. It will be almost as if we were working together in my office and you were working as my assistant on your own case.

Since foods, beverages, and food products are most often the culprits behind allergic arthritis (and many other disorders), you and I will first evaluate your possible food allergies.

Many patients who never suspected that their diet and their pattern of eating played even the slightest role in physical and/or mental-emotional disorders of long duration have been very surprised, even amazed, by the discoveries that we make in this area. The information we obtain from testing is often priceless—we may perform a few "miracles" together.

Carrying out the following instructions will provide you with a comprehensive list of the foods to which you are most likely to be allergic. It has been my experience and that of my colleagues that almost everyone—particularly those who are chronically afflicted— is allergic to something. Please be sure to prepare your information as accurately as possible. You are the only one who lives in and with this arthritic body of yours. *You* are the only one who can accurately draw this food-oriented clinical picture of yourself. Your body is unique biochemically and biologically; one of a kind; it is special and may very well respond to a given food in a manner that is different from that of anyone else.

Personal Diet Survey I

Using the form on pages 109–116, begin by making a checklist of those foods and beverages found in the average diet that you

1. Love and would be very upset about giving up.
2. Hate and avoid for whatever reason.
3. Have heavy exposure to and eat with great frequency
   a. at least one or more times a day.
   b. two to three times a week or more.
   c. very large amounts of once a week or more often.
4. Crave with some regularity—with a strong craving that no other food will satisfy; foods that are the object of binge eating.
5. Find especially satisfying for any reason, with a satisfaction or sense of well-being that goes beyond simple taste-bud enjoyment; foods that make you more alert, more energetic, stronger, re- laxed, or cause certain active symptoms to disappear or diminish in severity.

The foods and beverages you have placed on these lists may be important factors in your arthritis.

1. You may love a food because of its taste, but there are other important reasons (see items 4 and 5).
2. You may hate a food you are allergic to because, somehow, it disagrees with you very much and yet you are not sure of any specific reaction(s) it brings about. Or the hated food always makes you very ill. If you hate a particular food, this could be due to its odor or appearance, or there may be psychological factors associated with certain foods that have nothing to do with allergy

or addiction. In some instances hating a food is an important sign that this particular food allergically disagrees with you in a manner that is just below your threshold for developing definite recognizable symptoms. But it is most definitely doing something to you that identifies it as a very disagreeable substance, one that produces a reaction you are unable to describe properly. In a situation like this, hating a food is, to me, a very real symptom of food allergy.

3. Frequent intake of a given substance may push its level in your body to a point over your particular threshold of allergic tolerance, as I explained in Chapter 4. This food overload eventually leads to the appearance of a semipermanent, diet-sustained, cumulative allergic reaction that may smolder for years as low-level or moderate chronic symptoms. At times the chronic disorder may flare up in acute episodes of severe symptoms.

4. Cravings for certain foods may be manifestations of the addictive type of food allergy (see page 72). When the level of a food to which one has become addicted falls too low, this causes the symptoms of addictive withdrawal during which the food addict's allergic body "screams" for another "fix" of that food. Eating this food makes everything okay when you do not feel well because you have missed or were late for a meal containing the sympton-relieving food addictant.

5. Like most people, it is probable that you do not know why certain foods give you special satisfaction. For food-addicted allergic people, the ingestion of food to which they are sensitive will temporarily relieve their allergic-addictive withdrawal symptoms. Without realizing why, they turn to those favorite foods or beverages (alcoholic and nonalcoholic) over and over again—by habit or custom or deliberately—to make themselves feel better. This is the underlying cause of compulsive eating and compulsive alcoholic drinking.

Some highly addicted people who are eating offending foods very often have no idea that they even have a problem with addictive food allergy. Their specific food addictants never seem to cause trouble because the appearance of withdrawal symptoms is masked or blocked by the eating habits of these individuals. They consume their particular addicting dietary offenders before enough time has elapsed to permit the development of withdrawal symptoms, or they eat during the early phase of their food withdrawal reactions, which go unnoticed because they are so mild initially.

If a food definitely causes you to feel sick or if it makes some of your symptoms go away or decreases their severity, these changes constitute definite reactions—acute provocation of symptoms or neutralizing/masking symptom relief from the effects of an addicting food. Foods that you have observed to cause definite reactions recently or in the past are to be considered as probably offenders when diet testing is performed.

Based on the aforementioned information, you now understand why foods that you have checked in the first six columns of this first section of the Personal Diet Survey (I) belong on your list of probable or suspected arthritis-causing foods. Now go on to Section II of the Personal Diet Questionnaire.

Personal Diet Survey II—Your Exposure to Commonly Eaten Foods (Frequency of Ingestion)

In this section you will report your usual exposure to the foods that are eaten in the average diet. Place a mark (✓) in the appropriate column alongside the name of each food on the self-explanatory report form that starts on page 117. And be sure to check those foods that you eat in large quantities.

Personal Diet Survey

Section I

FEELINGS & RESPONSES

	ALL THESE FOODS ARE SUSPECT							Neutral* ? Safe ?
	Love	Hate	Crave	Binge	Feel Better	Feel Sick		
Acerola								
Alfalfa								
Almond								
American Cheese								

* The safety of "neutral" foods cannot be assumed because they appear to be tolerated. The role of each food must be established by testing (eating).

FEELINGS & RESPONSES

	ALL THESE FOODS ARE SUSPECT						Neutral* ? Safe ?
	Love	Hate	Crave	Binge	Feel Better	Feel Sick	
Anchovy							
Apple							
Apricot							
Arrowroot							
Artichoke Flour							
Asparagus							
Avocado							
Baker's Yeast							
Banana							
Barley							
Beef							
Beet							
Black Walnut							
Blueberry							
Bluefish							
Bran							
Brewer's Yeast							
Broccoli							

* The safety of "neutral" foods cannot be assumed because they appear to be tolerated. The role of each food must be established by testing (eating).

FEELINGS & RESPONSES

	ALL THESE FOODS ARE SUSPECT						
	Love	Hate	Crave	Binge	Feel Better	Feel Sick	Neutral* ? Safe?
Brussels Sprouts							
Buckwheat/Kasha							
Cabbage							
Cane Sugar							
Cantaloupe							
Caraway Seed							
Carob							
Carrot							
Cashew							
Cauliflower							
Celery							
Cheddar Cheese							
Cherry							
Chicken							
Chives							
Chocolate							
Cinnamon							
Clam							

* The safety of "neutral" foods cannot be assumed because they appear to be tolerated. The role of each food must be established by testing (eating).

FEELINGS & RESPONSES

	Love	Hate	Crave	Binge	Feel Better	Feel Sick	Neutral* ? Safe ?
ALL THESE FOODS ARE SUSPECT							
Cocoa							
Cod (Scrod)							
Cola							
Coffee							
Corn							
Crab							
Cranberry							
Cucumber							
Date							
Duck							
Egg							
Eggplant							
Flounder							
Garlic							
Grape/Raisins							
Grapefruit							
Haddock							
Halibut							

* The safety of "neutral" foods cannot be assumed because they appear to be tolerated. The role of each food must be established by testing (eating).

FEELINGS & RESPONSES

| | ALL THESE FOODS ARE SUSPECT | | | | | | Neutral* ? Safe ? |
	Love	Hate	Crave	Binge	Feel Better	Feel Sick	
Honey							
Honeydew							
Kidney Bean							
Lamb							
Lemon							
Lentil							
Lettuce							
Lobster							
Lima Bean							
Liver							
Mackerel							
Maple Syrup/Sugar							
Milk/Cottage Cheese							
Mushroom							
Mussel							
Mustard							
Navy Bean							
Oats							

* The safety of "neutral" foods cannot be assumed because they appear to be tolerated. The role of each food must be established by testing (eating).

FEELINGS & RESPONSES

	Love	Hate	Crave	Binge	Feel Better	Feel Sick	Neutral* ? Safe ?
	ALL THESE FOODS ARE SUSPECT						
Olive							
Onion							
Orange							
Pea							
Peach							
Peanut							
Pear							
Pecan							
Pepper, Black or White							
Pepper, Green							
Perch							
Pineapple							
Plum/Prune							
Pork/Ham/Bacon							
Potato							
Radish							
Rice							
Rye							

* The safety of "neutral" foods cannot be assumed because they appear to be tolerated. The role of each food must be established by testing (eating).

FEELINGS & RESPONSES

	ALL THESE FOODS ARE SUSPECT						Neutral*? Safe?
	Love	Hate	Crave	Binge	Feel Better	Feel Sick	
Red Snapper							
Safflower							
Salmon							
Scallops							
Shrimp							
Sole							
Soybean							
Spinach							
Squash							
Strawberry							
String Bean							
Sunflower Seed							
Sweet Potato							
Swiss Cheese							
Swordfish							
Tea							
Tomato							
Trout							

* The safety of "neutral" foods cannot be assumed because they appear to be tolerated. The role of each food must be established by testing (eating).

FEELINGS & RESPONSES

	ALL THESE FOODS ARE SUSPECT						Neutral* ? Safe ?
	Love	Hate	Crave	Binge	Feel Better	Feel Sick	
Tuna							
Turkey							
Turnip							
Vinegar							
Walnut							
Watermelon							
Wheat							
Yam							
Zucchini							

* The safety of "neutral" foods cannot be assumed because they appear to be tolerated. The role of each food must be established by testing (eating).

Personal Diet Survey

Section II

| | FREQUENCY OF INGESTION | | | | |
	Daily	2–3 Times a Week	Weekly	Every 2–4 Weeks	Large Portions
	SUSPECT	SUSPECT	POSSIBLE	UNLIKELY	SUSPECT
Acerola					
Alfalfa					
Almond					
American Cheese					
Anchovy					
Apple					
Apricot					
Arrowroot					
Artichoke Flour					
Asparagus					
Avocado					
Baker's Yeast					
Banana					
Barley					
Beef					
Beet					
Black Walnut					

	FREQUENCY OF INGESTION				
	Daily	2–3 Times a Week	Weekly	Every 2–4 Weeks	Large Portions
	SUSPECT	SUSPECT	POSSIBLE	UNLIKELY	SUSPECT
Blueberry					
Bluefish					
Bran					
Brewer's Yeast					
Broccoli					
Brussels Sprouts					
Buckwheat/Kasha					
Cabbage					
Cane Sugar					
Cantaloupe					
Caraway Seed					
Carob					
Carrot					
Cashew					
Cauliflower					
Celery					
Cheddar Cheese					
Cherry					
Chicken					

| | FREQUENCY OF INGESTION | | | | |
| | Daily | 2–3 Times a Week | Weekly | Every 2–4 Weeks | Large Portions |
	SUSPECT	SUSPECT	POSSIBLE	UNLIKELY	SUSPECT
Chives					
Chocolate					
Cinnamon					
Clam					
Cocoa					
Cod (Scrod)					
Cola					
Coffee					
Corn					
Crab					
Cranberry					
Cucumber					
Date					
Duck					
Egg					
Eggplant					
Flounder					
Garlic					
Grape/Raisin					

	FREQUENCY OF INGESTION				
	Daily	2–3 Times a Week	Weekly	Every 2–4 Weeks	Large Portions
	SUSPECT	SUSPECT	POSSIBLE	UNLIKELY	SUSPECT
Grapefruit					
Haddock					
Halibut					
Honey					
Honeydew					
Kidney Bean					
Lamb					
Lemon					
Lentil					
Lettuce					
Lobster					
Lima Bean					
Liver					
Mackerel					
Maple Syrup/Sugar					
Milk/Cottage Cheese					
Mushroom					
Mussel					
Mustard					

| | FREQUENCY OF INGESTION | | | | |
	Daily	2–3 Times a Week	Weekly	Every 2–4 Weeks	Large Portions
	SUSPECT	SUSPECT	POSSIBLE	UNLIKELY	SUSPECT
Navy Bean					
Oats					
Olive					
Onion					
Orange					
Pea					
Peach					
Peanut					
Pear					
Pecan					
Pepper, Black or White					
Pepper, Green					
Perch					
Pineapple					
Plum/Prune					
Pork/Ham/Bacon					
Potato					
Radish					
Rice					

| | FREQUENCY OF INGESTION | | | | |
	Daily	2–3 Times a Week	Weekly	Every 2–4 Weeks	Large Portions
	SUSPECT	SUSPECT	POSSIBLE	UNLIKELY	SUSPECT
Rye					
Red Snapper					
Safflower					
Salmon					
Scallops					
Shrimp					
Sole					
Soybean					
Spinach					
Squash					
Strawberry					
String Bean					
Sunflower Seed					
Sweet Potato					
Swiss Cheese					
Swordfish					
Tea					
Tomato					
Trout					

| | FREQUENCY OF INGESTION | | | | |
	Daily	2–3 Times a Week	Weekly	Every 2–4 Weeks	Large Portions
	SUSPECT	SUSPECT	POSSIBLE	UNLIKELY	SUSPECT
Tuna					
Turkey					
Turnip					
Vinegar					
Walnut					
Watermelon					
Wheat					
Yam					
Zucchini					

Diagnosis of Probable Food Allergy Based on Reactions to Alcoholic Beverages

Acute reactions to alcoholic beverages, or "morning after" hangovers (delayed withdrawal symptoms), strongly indicate the possibility of food allergy to the food source materials from which the symptom-causing alcoholic drink is produced.

Some otherwise nonreaction-causing foods that are eaten along with an alcoholic beverage may also cause reactions. Foods involved in such reactions are potential dietary offenders. They become "activated"—a food-overdose effect occurs as the foods are very rapidly absorbed into the circulation in the ethyl alcohol "solvent." Mixed with alcohol, innocent foods can easily become allergic troublemakers. The same foods may be well tolerated if they are eaten without ingesting an alcoholic beverage—the allergic threshold level for the potential allergens is not exceeded, and no symptoms appear if there is no alcohol present to accelerate the absorption rate of the food.

Alcoholic beverages are made by the yeast fermentation of natural sugars in sugar-containing foods (grapes, apples, etc.) and from sugars that are released from the enzymatic breakdown of starch present in starch-containing cereal grains and foods. For example, rum is made from cane sugar; sake from rice; beer and bourbon by converting cornstarch to corn sugar (glucose or dextrose), which is then fermented. Potato starch is the source of Russian vodka and Swedish aquavit; grape sugar of wine, rye of rye whiskey*, and barley of Scotch whiskey.

Source material from the original grain, vegetable, or fruit is present, and often allergically active, in the final product—the yeast-fermented alcoholic beverage.

Reactions to mixed drinks may be caused by the sugar and/or lemon in a whiskey sour, the tomato or spices in a Bloody Mary, or the orange juice in a screwdriver. These food ingredients are rapidly absorbed when they are present in an alcoholic vehicle.

Some of the common allergic reactions to alcohol are: rashes, itching, bloating, gas, indigestion, abdominal cramps, nausea, facial swelling, puffy eyelids, nasal congestion, cough, headache, visual

---

*The designation "rye whiskey" can be confusing, since the word *rye* is often used to identify various blended whiskeys manufactured from several types of grain. The alcoholic beverage that is derived solely from the fermentation and distillation of rye grain is the beverage referred to herein. As far as I know, Canadian rye is a 100% rye product.

REACTIONS TO ALCOHOLIC DOSAGES

	Immediate	Within an hour	Next morning	Symptoms noted
Applejack				
Beer				
Bourbon				
Brandy				
Gin mixture				
Liqueurs				
Rum mixture				
Rye				
Scotch mix				
Vermouth mix				
Vodka				
Blended whiskey				
Canadian whiskey				
Wine				
Bloody Mary				
Manhattan				
Martini				
Screwdriver				
Whiskey sour				

Foods Used in Preparation of Alcoholic Beverages

	GRAINS							POTATO	FRUITS									MISCELLANEOUS							SUGAR, YEAST, WATER			
	Corn (a)	Barley (malt) (b)	Rye (c)	Wheat (d)	Oats	Rice	Milo (e)	Potato	Grape	Plum	Citrus	Apple	Pear	Apricot	Peach	Cherry	Berries	Carob	Hops	Juniper	Cinnamon	Mint	Miscl. Herbs	Cactus	Beet (f)	Cane (f)	Yeast (g)	Water
WHISKY Straight Corn	●	●	●	○	○	○	○																				●	●
" Bourbon	●	●	●	○	○	○	○																				●	●
" Malt	●	●	●	○	○	○	○																				●	●
" Rye	●	●	●	○	○	○	○																				●	●
" Wheat	●	●	○	●	○	○	○																				●	●
Blended Straight Corn	●	●	●	○	○	●	○																				●	●
" " Bourbon	●	●	●	○	○	●	○																				●	●
" " Malt	●	●	●	○	○	●	○																				●	●
" " Rye	●	●	●	○	○	●	○																				●	●
" " Rye-malt	●	●	●	○	○	●	○																				●	●
" " Wheat	●	●	○	●	○	●	○																				●	●
Blended	●	●	●	○	○	○	○	○	○	○	○	○	○	○	○	○	○	○									●	●
Light	●	●	●	○	○	○	○	○	○	○	○	○	○	○	○	○	○	○							●	●	●	●
Spirit	●	●	○	○	○	○	○	○			○														●	●	●	●
*Canadian (Blended)	●	●	●	●					●	●	○														○	●	●	●

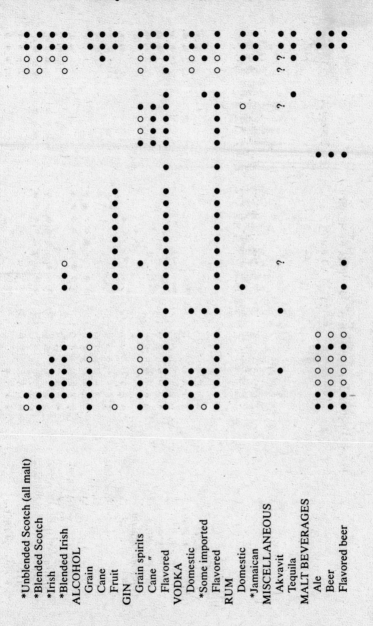

*Unblended Scotch (all malt)
*Blended Scotch
*Irish
*Blended Irish
ALCOHOL
  Grain
  Cane
  Fruit
GIN
  Grain spirits
  Cane "
  Flavored
VODKA
  Domestic
*Some imported
  Flavored
RUM
  Domestic
*Jamaican
MISCELLANEOUS
  Akvavit
  Tequila
MALT BEVERAGES
  Ale
  Beer
  Flavored beer

	GRAINS				POTATO	FRUITS									MISCELLANEOUS						SUGAR, YEAST, WATER				
	Corn	Barley-Rye-Wheat	Oats	Rice	Potato	Grape	Plum	Citrus	Apple	Pear	Apricot	Peach	Cherry	Berries	Juniper	Coconut	Cinnamon	Chocolate	Mint	Miscl. Herbs	Honey	Beet	Cane	Yeast	Water
BRANDY																									
Grape	○					●																○	○	●	●
Raisin	○					●																○	○	●	●
Cognac						●																○	○	●	●
Plum	○						●															○	○	●	●
Applejack	○								●													○	○	●	●
Apricot	○										●											○	○	●	●
Peach	○											●										○	○	●	●
Cherry	○												●									○	○	●	●
Blackberry	○													●								○	○	●	●
Fruit	○					●	●	●	●	●	●	●	●	●								○	○	●	●
Neutral	○																					○	○	●	●
*Juniper															●							?	?		●
FRUIT FLAVORED BRANDY	●	●	○	○	○	●	●	●	●	●	●	●	●	●		○	●	●	●	●	○	●	●	●	●
CORDIALS AND LIQUEURS	●	●	○	○	○	●	●	●	●	●	●	●	●	●		○	●	●	●	●	○	●	●	●	●

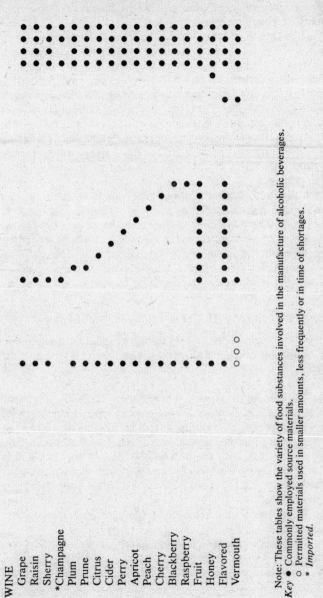

WINE
Grape
Raisin
Sherry
*Champagne
Plum
Prune
Citrus
Cider
Perry
Apricot
Peach
Cherry
Blackberry
Raspberry
Fruit
Honey
Flavored
Vermouth

Note: These tables show the variety of food substances involved in the manufacture of alcoholic beverages.

Key ● Commonly employed source materials.
○ Permitted materials used in smaller amounts, less frequently or in time of shortages.
* Imported.

Reprinted from "The Role of Specific Alcoholic Beverages," by Theron G. Randolph, M.D., in Clinical Ecology, ed. L. D. Dickey, M.D. (Springfield, Ill.: Charles C. Thomas, Publisher, 1976), pp. 326 and 329.

blurring, depression, nervousness, dizziness, fatigue, joint and muscle pains, and body soreness.

Now it is time to review carefully the foods in the three lists you have just completed—your responses to the frequency with which you eat each of them. If there is any food that you may have overlooked—one that you can associate with any kind of possible allergic reaction now or in the past—be certain that there is a check mark indicating this fact. For instance, you may suddenly recall that you often get heartburn after eating tuna fish or can taste and retaste it many hours later. Or, reviewing your past, you remember breaking out in a nasty, itching, generalized rash after gorging on strawberries as a child. You might discuss this with your parents or an older brother or sister.

When you perform your series of deliberate food ingestion tests outlined in the next chapters, you will begin by testing your number-one suspects. This will include all the foods that caused symptoms, relieved symptoms, were craved or binged on, loved or loaded up on, or appear in the common-offenders on page 155. These are the prime suspects for your arthritis, but there may be a few surprises awaiting you among some of the seemingly benign items in your diet.

Personal Diet Survey III—Your Prime Suspect List

Before you begin your self-help testing program, let's make one more search for additional diagnostic clues that may be at your fingertips.

> Think about the times you have gone without eating on your usual schedule. Perhaps it was because of an extrabusy school or office schedule, or during a religious fast day. It might have been when you were on a very restricted crash diet or when you were too sick with the intestinal flu bug to feel like eating anything. At those times of decreased food exposure, has your arthritis improved? If so, it is very likely that your arthritis *is* food related.
>
> When you miss a meal, what foods or beverages do you crave?
>
> What foods make you feel better if missing a meal makes you ill?
>
> When your normal diet is drastically altered, what foods, if any, do you crave?

Does a drastic change in diet relieve or increase symptoms that you can then associate with eating or eliminating any particular foods?

What foods have you ever associated with an improvement in your arthritis?

What foods do you associate with making your arthritis worse?

Do any alcoholic beverages relieve your arthritis immediately or overnight, and what foods are they made from?

Do any alcoholic beverages either cause or aggravate attacks of arthritic symptoms? What are they made from?

The foods identified by the answers to those questions certainly must be on your list of suspects when you begin to test yourself for food allergies as you read the next chapter.

If you have done your best and still have important questions that remain unanswered, and you can't find the answers in my other books (see pp. 261–263), my staff and I will try to help. You may write to me at the address on page 257. Make your question(s) simple so I can write yes or no, or give me a choice of answers so I will be able to circle, check, or underline the correct one. Do everything to make it easy for me to give you a prompt reply and you will receive one. Send a self-addressed, stamped envelope, and I will return my answer on your original letter.

I will try to help, but I cannot be your personal physician. I cannot prescribe for you. You must obtain additional information about medications and the like from your pharmacist or your personal doctor.

7

How to Free Your System from Arthritis-Causing Substances

You are now almost ready to test yourself for the presence of food allergies that may be causing your arthritis and, perhaps, other important physical and/or mental conditions. For your self-testing to be as accurate as possible, you must first rid your body of (or greatly reduce) the residue of all the arthritis-provoking food offenders you have been eating during the past few months. In most instances these will be the same foods that you have been eating for many years. Clearing your system of clinically important residues of the specific food allergens that have been causing chronic or recurrent arthritic reactions in your joints and muscles will result in certain bodily changes. These internal changes will make it possible for you to provoke acute flare-ups of your chronic arthritis by means of a series of self-administered Rinkel deliberate food (feeding) tests (DFTs) that are of great diagnostic value.

Dr. Herbert Rinkel, one of the pioneering allergists whose many research findings helped establish the field of clinical ecology, observed that if an allergenic food causing chronic symptoms is eliminated from the diet for a period of time ranging from four to twelve days or longer (up to eighteen to twenty-one days in some individuals), a patient will become highly sensitive (hyperreactive) to that food during the elimination period after the fourth day and will remain so up to two or three weeks thereafter. When it is reintroduced to the diet during the hyperreactive state, it will cause an acute, diagnostically important flare-up of the familiar chronic symptoms that were previously caused by the offending food.

This chapter details procedures for two offending-food-removal techniques from which you may choose. They are the Food Elimination Diet and the Spring Water Fast. Each method will take from five to seven days.

During the process of digestion the foods you eat are broken down into their basic chemical components, which may be used immediately, may be stored in cells throughout your body, and/or may remain in the blood or the extracellular fluid that surrounds body cells. Clinical experience has shown that it usually takes four to five days or longer for the body's natural biochemical processes (metabolism) to break down or excrete the unused or unneeded fractions of those stored, food-derived basic chemicals, either removing them from the system or bringing them well below the allergic threshold level.

My Food Elimination Diet accomplishes its objective because, as we clinical ecologists have found, a group of commonly eaten foods—which are included in almost every diet—are among the most important causes of the many kinds of internal allergic disorders.

The most frequently identified food offenders—the most often consumed, illness-causing foods—are: wheat and other members of the grass family such as corn, oats, rye, rice, and cane sugar. The other major offenders are milk, eggs, beef, yeast, soy, chicken, pork, apples, green beans, oranges, bananas, potatoes, lettuce, tomatoes, carrots, peanuts, coffee, tea, and chocolate (cocoa).

By having you follow a diet that omits all the aforementioned foods and consists of only those foods that are not eaten as often, you are much less likely to have the allergic joint and muscle reactions of arthritis. Reactions will be even less likely if these uncommon foods are eaten in a carefully planned rotation (rotary) diet that prevents a reaction-evoking buildup of any potential dietary offender in your system.

In order to prevent any error on your part, let us review the basic principles of this stage of your self-help program. You will start by eliminating those common foods to which you may be allergic because they have been eaten too frequently for many years. In addition, you will also eliminate all or most of the other possible illness evoking foods, because of your personal food habits and your observations regarding their known or suspected effects on your health. The Food Elimination Diet automatically eliminates many active, probable, and potential arthritis-evoking allergens.

The dietary rotation of less frequently consumed foods rapidly frees the system of the residual effects of previous meals that contained the more frequently ingested foods that were, in all probability, causing allergic joint reactions.

It is possible for you to get away with it for a while by eating in an unplanned manner. However, I urge you to avoid an unnecessary waste of time and effort—and possible disappointment—by carefully following a rotary diversified diet that eliminates or at least greatly reduces the possibility of poor or fair results that often come from easily preventable cumulative reactions. The buildup of illness-evoking components present in arthritis-causing foods is controlled by ingesting potential offenders on a schedule that permits the body to recover from the initial presymptom effects of a given food before it is eaten again. You must eat the uncommon foods in a well-planned rotation that preserves your existing tolerance to these foods (and also prevents the symptoms that would have come from the ingestion of common food offenders) by employing the Rinkel Rotary Diversified Diet technique that I discuss beginning on page 154.

All you have to do is eat three different, unspiced, unflavored (except for the use of sea salt) single-food meals each day, with a different food at every meal. The foods eaten each day should be carefully selected and arranged from different food families in a way that prevents the buildup of a family-specific substance that may be present in the different members of a closely related group of foods. (Food families are discussed beginning on page 157.) Cumulative reactions of this type are usually avoided by alternate-day spacing of exposures to food-family members like orange and grapefruit, carrot and celery, apple and pear, and so on. The five-, six-, or seven-day cycle of every rotation diet should be repeated several times with each new selection of foods, making it possible for you to record and recheck your observations of the reproducible effects of individual foods. The foods are eaten in a controlled manner, following a period of avoidance, that unmasks food addiction and provokes familiar symptoms that clearly demonstrate the causal relationship of these dietary factors in your arthritis (as well as any other allergy-related health problems you may have).

It is possible that a perfectly planned and perfectly followed rotary diet may not help very much—or not at all—in a food-allergic arthritic person who has other serious allergies. This unhappy situation results because there is a massive chemical or inhalant-allergen overload in the environment that is so great it will not allow any relief to appear even if the food-allergic arthritic person were completely to control food exposure by fasting. The nonfood offenders independently overwhelm the chemically susceptible, inhalant-sensitive patient—they constitute a massive exposure that elicits a maximal symptom response. If there is a bad "chemical problem," it will cause symptoms even though the foods are very well controlled, and vice versa.

Examples of just a few environmental factors that may be responsible for this kind of problem include the following:

1. Airborne allergens that the arthritis sufferer is extremely sensitive to are inhaled, absorbed into the circulation, transported to the active or potentially active arthritis sites, and cause flare-ups. They include tree, grass, and weed pollens; indoor and outdoor molds; animal dander; house dust, dust mites, and insect particles.
2. Biologically reactive chemical substances like ammonia, formaldehyde and chlorine; coal tar and petrochemically derived substances that are added to foods and are used in pharmaceutical preparations.
3. Petrochemical fumes arise from fuels, combustion products, solvents, perfumes, wax, paints, disinfectants, tars, plastics, permanent markers, hair spray, deodorants, and a leaking gas stove.
4. Tobacco smoke is a very complex mixture that has combustion fumes from tobacco, chemically treated paper, and numerous chemicals that are used on tobacco crops and by the tobacco industry during the manufacturing process.

Several years ago a young Canadian housewife came to me to be tested for "chemicals and molds" because she *knew* that foods were not important in her case. She came to this conclusion because she had fasted for six days and saw no improvement in her headache, fatigue, digestive, and respiratory complaints as well as her joint and muscle pains. She had a gas stove in the kitchen, her home was heated with a gas hot-air system, she used a variety of the usual household chemicals, the basement was damp and had a distinct mildew odor, and her husband was a cigarette smoker.

Our comprehensive diagnostic studies included symptom-duplicating, provocative sublingual tests for food allergy in addition to the sublingual and inhalation tests for inhalant allergies and chemical susceptibility that she had requested. She was correct regarding her self-diagnosis of internal (systemic) allergies to several species of mold as well as weed pollens, and she also reacted to chemical provocation testing with petroleum alcohol, tobacco smoke, chlorine, and natural gas.

She was completely wrong about her moderately severe food allergies. She had overlooked them entirely because her at-home fasting was done in a moldy, chemically polluted environment. The molds and chemicals in her home affected her so much that they independently caused important symptoms during her fasting period, which totally freed her from all the symptoms caused by foods and diverted her attention from the important role of dietary factors in a complex situation that involved a clinically significant degree of allergic sensitivity to foods as well as to both inhalants and chemicals.

It is difficult for me to understand the thinking of conventional allergists who insist that food allergies are not very common or particularly important. Pollen allergy is the cause of eye and respiratory disorders that they really "believe in," but it seems to me that they have not paid enough attention to what pollens actually are—concentrated particles of plant (vegetable) material that cause symptoms when they contact the surface of the eyes or enter the respiratory tract. Similarly, the molds the conventional allergists work with daily are very simple life forms that maintain themselves by ingesting and incorporating within themselves the substances comprising the various plant and animal foods eaten by humans. And allergically potent animal dander responsible for the misery of many allergy victims is composed of the skin flakes of animals like hogs and cattle that are major sources of the meat people consume. The obvious relationship between foods that my ecologically oriented colleagues and I recognize as major allergens and the conventional allergists' "overworked" pollens, molds, and dander are important facts that need to be given serious consideration, and another clinically valuable perspective will have been gained.

Read through both the Spring Water Fast and The Food Elimination Diet plans carefully and decide which you prefer to follow. Whichever plan you choose, there is an excellent chance that you will make some important discoveries regarding the effects of food on your arthritis as well as on your health in general.

You may decide that, being in good condition otherwise, you want to employ the fasting technique simultaneously to eliminate all the possible adverse effects from food and food technology and perhaps lose some weight at the same time. This is fine with me, but a physical examination, routine blood and urine tests and the *approval of your physician* are necessary. *Take no unnecessary risks* with your health.

If you are in reasonably good health, there should be no serious difficulty regarding fasting. *Follow your physician's advice regarding medications* currently being taken and be sure to drink at least six to eight glasses of bottled-in-glass spring or well water daily. And do not forget that you may develop withdrawal symptoms as foods you are addicted to begin to show the power of allergic addiction.

In some fasting patients, for whom multiple factors are responsible for their arthritis, there may be a temporary improvement and even very great relief of arthritis and other symptoms for a short period of time. For a little while the allergic body reacts favorably because some major food offenders have been eliminated. The reduction in the total load of allergic stresses provides a much-needed biologic rest period. But the beneficial effects of fasting may be short-lived in some instances, because the combined effects of other uncontrolled ecologic factors may bring about a gradual return of symptoms.

However, you can be very optimistic if this happens to you, because you will have proved that *you actually were able temporarily to reverse the chronic arthritic process* using only some of the bioecologic self-help that is available. You did not employ any drug to obtain this natural relief, which you achieved by means of a relatively simple control measure involving one aspect of your environmental-dietary allergic illness.

If your arthritic symptoms do not improve, you may still be a victim of food allergy, but you will also know that "chemicals" and/ or inhalants are likely offenders even if your answers to the questionnaires regarding responses to native airborne allergens and various chemical agents did not suggest that they are factors in your illness.

If you would like to lose some weight but do not wish to fast, you can reduce your caloric intake and use some of your unwanted body-fat deposits as an energy source by eating either one or two single-food test meals per day. Each day be sure that you have one high-protein food like meat, poultry or fish.* These protein-rich foods

---

*In order to spare muscle tissue and internal organs and to provide for repair of normal tissue breakdown as well as supplying necessary structural building materials for your cells and components for hormones and enzymes, etc., it is suggested that you consume at least 8 ounces of a high-protein food each day. Protein foods supply a needed material for body maintenance; you certainly do not want to have some of your tissues broken down to supply what is missing from your diet if you are not on a fast.

should be ones that you do not eat very often. Here is a golden opportunity to indulge in my medically prescribed special menu of "exotic" lobster, duck, king crab, pheasant, rabbit, turtle, venison, squab, frog's legs, wild rice, palm cabbage, macadamia nuts, pistachio nuts, persimmons, mango, artichoke, water chestnuts, papaya, cactus pears—whatever happens to tickle your fancy.

You will learn whether your food allergy is fixed, cyclic, or addictive (see pp. 70–74). Those with addictive food allergies will experience withdrawal symptoms on the first, second, or third day of the Food Elimination Diet or during fasting. Arthritis may flare up dramatically and, because allergies usually affect other systems in cases of arthritis, you may also experience some nonarthritic symptoms like stomach cramps, mental confusion, restlessness, fatigue, headache, itching, sweating, or flulike symptoms; some individuals may strongly crave a particular food. These withdrawal reactions occur when the level of the "food chemical" to which the body is addicted falls below a certain point and the addicted body send out a sort of SOS for another "dose" or "fix" of the addicting food. The SOS is broadcast throughout the body of the food addict in the form of uncomfortable withdrawal symptoms that are usually generalized. Methods of treating the manifestations of this withdrawal phase are fully discussed elsewhere in this book. If you do not experience any withdrawal symptoms and find that your arthritis has been relieved by the special diet or fasting, you will know that you have just cleared up a fixed food allergy or a cumulative cyclic food allergy.

A Very Important Personal Message

Some readers may initially react both to the diet and the fast with comments such as, "This is too complicated" or "I could never manage that!" To them I say, "Read and reread this part of my book a few times, and I know that you will appreciate the beautiful logic and fundamental simplicity of this almost-foolproof self-help method of diagnosing arthritis that is caused by serious food allergies. This commonsense way to relieve your arthritis will cost nothing beyond the price of this book and the foods that you eat. And there is an excellent chance that you will be able to improve your health without the use of drugs and their avoidable side effects. Is it worth a few minutes a day for just a few days of your time—some effort and a little inconvenience—to be able to rid yourself of the pain and stiffness that now limit your physical activities and affect the quality of your entire life? And may lead to greater, now preventable, future disability? Think about it, and the answer has to be yes.

WE are going to fight this misery together. The odds are strongly in our favor that we will identify and eliminate or gain control over the causes of your arthritis. We shall overcome!

The only people for whom fasting could possibly cause more potential harm than good are a small group of individuals who have serious medical or psychological problems that might be adversely affected by fasting. Get your doctor's advice and a checkup before fasting. If your doctor says that you are physically able to fast, and you want to do so but are apprehensive, for whatever reason, about the possible effects of fasting, you could fast in a hospital under the supervision of a physician who is familiar with fasting. There are some very complex and serious cases, beyond the scope of an ecologist's office practice, that will require admission to an environmentally controlled ecologic unit.

No matter which method you use to remove arthritis-causing food residues from your system, you should follow these general guidelines.

> *Make your environment as ecologically "clean" as possible.* Some patients have written, telephoned, or come to my office complaining that they fasted on spring water without cheating but saw no improvement whatsoever in return for their serious efforts. In those cases it turned out that most of the patients really were allergic to foods—very allergic, in many instances—but they also were sensitive to various chemicals and/ or airborne inhalant allergens that had not been eliminated from or sufficiently reduced in the home environment. You probably cannot completely remove *all* the potential arthritis-evoking chemical and inhalant offenders from your home and place of employment, but you can go a long way toward the creation of an almost ideal environment by the following steps. For a working person, it would be a great help if you could be on vacation or sick leave, thereby avoiding many exposures.

1. Turn off all gas appliances (cook on an electric double-burner hot plate and electric oven-broiler, heat with an electric heater, and hang your laundry outdoors to dry if you have a gas dryer. Do not use a kerosene heater or propane-fueled equipment.

2. If your garage is part of your house—not connected by a breeze-way—remove from it all the chemicals and the fuel-operated equipment like cars, motorcycles and lawn mowers, etc.

3. For bedding, use only pure, untreated cotton. Since most pillows are filled with synthetics or feathers, you should avoid them. Instead, stuff a cotton pillowcase with cotton towels. Do not use an odorous synthetic "nonallergic" pillow or mattress cover. Allergy-free or allergen-proof casings for pillows and mattresses can cause important symptoms in allergic patients who are chemically susceptible. In fact, the chemical allergies may be more severe than the dust and cotton or feather allergy symptoms that the casings are "protecting" the patients from.

4. Be certain that no tobacco smoke or chemical agents that produce odors or vapors, such as paints, furniture polish, floor wax, air fresheners, chlorine-releasing cleansers, laundry bleach and detergents, insect sprays, disinfectants, etc., are used in your home during your fast. Consider this to be one of those rare prescriptions to have all the housekeeping activities come to a temporary halt.

5. Avoid scented substances like soaps, shampoos, hair sprays, deodorants, perfumes, colognes, skin bracers, aftershave and preshave lotions, and all other cosmetics. If you have any doubt about exposing yourself to something, do not use it.

6. Have a collection of recreational materials on hand. But be sure they're old, and thoroughly air out books, magazines, games, and cards before using them. Newer materials of this kind may contain active chemicals that are released into the surrounding air.

7. Board your pets, with their dander, saliva, and body odors, and board your plants, with their mold-containing soil, because they too should be away from your home at this time.

Remember, fasting means exactly what it says—no food or beverages at all, and that includes very weak tea and diluted fruit or vegetable juices. This also means no coffee (including de-caf), herbal teas, alcohol, soda, or tap water. You are to ingest *only* spring water or untreated well water, salted to taste with sea salt or kosher salt, if desired. Many fasting patients are pleasantly surprised to find that a cup of hot spring water is just as satisfying as their usual hot beverages. The sight of a steaming teapot with its matching cup and saucer has pleased many fasting people.

Smoking by you and by others in your home is forbidden. Don't panic at this rule, even if you consider yourself a hopeless nicotine addict! Time after time patients have reported that giving up their tobacco habit was extraordinarily easy for them while fasting. It's really the best time to eliminate a very important offender and protect your overall health from the long-term noxious effects of smoking.

Keep a careful daily record of the observations you make concerning reactions during your fast, using a form like that on pages 151–153. It is especially important to note any flare-ups of your arthritis as well as the appearance of any other familiar physical or mental symptoms. These are the withdrawal reactions of food allergy that usually occur on the second or third day of a fast, but they may appear during the first day in some instances. They are very good signs that you should welcome, because they almost guarantee that some food or foods in your usual diet are capable of causing addictive withdrawal reactions. Your body is telling you that addictive food allergy is an important factor in the causation of your allergic arthritis—and other health problems. (Should your food-induced symptoms cause a moderate to severe degree of discomfort, try one of the remedies listed on pages 149–150 to obtain relief.) Any cravings you may have are significant, too, because an uncontrollable biologic need for a particular food, until proven otherwise, is pointing directly to other offending dietary substances that affect your health in some way.

Write it all down in detail. Do not trust your memory. That severe, dramatic, and interesting reaction you may experience with great surprise on a particular day—the one you are certain you will never forget—will soon blend with the impressive food-provoked reactions of the following days. And if you are like many of my patients, within a few days to a week, it will be impossible for you to remember clearly just what happened after eating a particular food on a certain day. There will almost certainly be some areas of confusion about some test responses as a result of your failure to keep adequate records. All is not lost, however, if this happens, because you can always retest yourself to confirm your findings—and even show your doubting relatives and friends and just possibly teach your doctor something very important about the chronic joint disease without a "known" cause or a "curative" method of treatment.

The Five-Day Spring Water Fast

The word *fast* turns some people off because they wonder if they can possibly go without eating. Let me clear up some possible misunderstandings. Contrary to the beliefs of some, five days or longer of total fasting is not absolutely essential to rid the body of all food offenders or to decrease their residual effects to clinically undetectable levels.

In my own office practice less than three percent of the patients I see are fully fasted by ingesting only spring water for five days. On occasion a patient requests my assistance with a voluntary fast, and I cooperate when it is in the patient's best interest. In carefully selected, severe cases of environmental-allergic illness, it may be necessary or much easier on the patient—especially one who lives alone—to do this in the ecologic unit of a hospital that is under the continuous, direct supervision of one of my fellow ecologists and his staff.

Fasting can be the quickest and most effective approach, because within a few days—less than one week—it shows how much of your illness is a reversible disorder caused by food allergy and environmental sensitivity. It is wonderful to know that your arthritis can be controlled completely when your diet is totally changed to pure water in a nonpolluted and allergen-free environment. Fasting and environmental control can provide you with a dramatic demonstration of how much better you can feel as soon as the allergens are removed from your system, as these cases of Dr. Harris Hosen, of Port Arthur, Texas, illustrate.

A patient with rheumatoid arthritis as well as bronchial and nasal allergies was completely relieved of all respiratory and arthritic symptoms after four days on a spring-water fast.

A sixty-five-year-old woman lost all her multiple allergy symptoms, including arthritis, during a 5½-day fast.

Another woman had unexplainable and incurable gastrointestinal symptoms despite ten years of ineffective special diets, blood and urine testing, X rays, sigmoidoscopy, and many drug treatments. She also had severe arthritic aches and pains. Her severe unsuspected and undetected food allergies led to a diagnosis of "neuroses." Happily, she was cleared of all symptoms after 4½ days of fasting! After ten years of unnecessary illness it was absolutely gone, without any drugs, exposure to radiation, laboratory expenses, or discomfort.

The spring-water fast is not nearly as difficult as you may imagine. In fact, the rules are quite simple. You avoid taking into your system anything but bottled untreated spring water, which, unlike tap water, contains no reactive chemical agents like chlorine, fluoride, manufacturing wastes, and the "runoff" of agricultural chemicals from the soil and crops that is carried by rain and melting snow to the local water supply.

In addition to the environmental precautions listed on pages 140–141, prepare for your fast by stocking up on bottled-in-glass spring water. Keep in mind that most fasting patients drink one or two quarts or more each day. You will probably use between three and four gallons for drinking, brushing your teeth, and rinsing your mouth during the fast. Some adjustment upward may be required during the summer. The "relief" substances for making your fast as comfortable as possible are listed on pages 149–150 and should be obtained. If possible, clear your home of whatever might become a source of tantalizing odors, such as open containers of food. Tell family and friends of your plan to fast and what is required of them with respect to smoking, cosmetics, and the like.

Pick a good day to begin your fast. For instance, if you work from Monday to Friday, start on a Thursday evening by drinking only spring water at suppertime. In that way you will be off work during Saturday and Sunday, the days you are most likely to experience withdrawal symptoms.

For five days ingest *nothing* but glass-bottled spring water. Take no vitamins or nonessential medications. Review all your medications with your doctor and take only those that you cannot get along without. Use no toothpaste or mouthwash (brush with sea salt or baking soda and use unwaxed dental floss) or just massage your gums with your toothbrush. Don't take even a single sip of tap water. Don't smoke, chew gum, or drink tea or coffee. Do not use cologne, aftershave lotion, or perfumed soap.

Drink *lots* of spring water, hot or cold. You may use spring-water ice cubes. You need at least six to eight full glasses daily, preferably more, to keep your kidneys and intestines functioning well and to help them eliminate the wastes and stored chemicals from your body.

Exercise gently; walk, do yoga, stretch. Get as much rest and sleep as you can. Maintain as even a temperature as possible, avoiding extreme heat or cold.

Take a mild laxative every two to three days, and if necessary for constipation or discomfort, take an enema. Those I recommend are listed on pages 149–150. My current instructions for an at-home fast include citrate magnesia the first evening and a sodium bicarbonate enema the following morning.

If withdrawal symptoms make you uncomfortable, use one of the relieving measures on pages 149–150. If you experience any severe symptoms that cause you concern, contact your physician. In fact, make sure he knows about your fasting in advance so you will not surprise him. Remember that prefasting physical examination you should have.

Although you may feel hunger during the first day and perhaps a little longer, that sensation will disappear shortly as your body calls on its stored energy reserves. Many people find that on a fast they feel better physically and mentally—that they are more alert and more satisfied with life in general than they usually are.

Keep careful records on a form like the one on pages 151–153. (This form is suitable for fasting patients as well as those who are eating.) Remember that withdrawal symptoms indicate the presence of an addictive food allergy that is in the process of clearing up. The energy that is released from the metabolism of one-half pound of your stored fat reserves is all that you need each day during your fast, and a five-day fast will only require about three pounds from this energy reserve. You may lose much more weight in the form of water.

Many allergic people retain fluid because allergic reactions in their thin-walled capillary blood vessels allow fluid to leak from the circulation into their tissues. There may be some allergic changes in the kidneys that could also cause some water retention. It is not unusual for patients to lose from three to five pounds or more of retained water as the capillaries, and perhaps the kidneys, return to normal when exposure to allergens stops. Puffy eyelids, lips, hands, and feet (with tight rings and tight shoes) may clear up unexpectedly.

Some people who do not look the least puffy may lose five or more pounds, because the retained fluid may have been evenly distributed throughout the body. I have seen some trim-looking patients who did not seem the least bit overweight lose significant amounts of weight this way. This, of course, explains why a person who does not have heart or kidney disease may be taking "water pills" to control weight; the doctor doesn't know about allergic water retention, a condition that requires no pills when the allergic problem is brought under control.

Dr. Hosen introduced me to one of his hospital patients in Texas about ten years ago. She had three completely different wardrobes because she needed three different sizes of clothing, depending on where she was in her twenty-five-pound weight range, which shifted from one extreme to the other over two- to three-day periods for a number of years. On her plus-twenty-five days, people who knew her on her minus-twenty-five-days did not even recognize her because of her general appearance and the striking changes in her facial features. During her fast in St. Mary's Hospital in Beaumont, Texas, she lost her usual twenty-five pounds and felt great—alive, alert and energetic; her rings fit, she wore her smallest shoes and smallest-size clothing. Her condition was controlled by avoidance of the fluid-retaining food allergens that were identified by Dr. Hosen.

The following case of "chemical arthritis" is presented in detail because it will give my readers a great deal of very interesting information about fasting, comprehensive environmental control, and ecologic diagnosis and treatment.

A sixty-one-year-old man living in Indiana, Charles Voors was incapacitated by arthritis caused by an allergylike sensitivity to chemicals in his total environment. He is an excellent example of a serious case of food-related chemical susceptibility associated with susceptibility to atmospheric chemical fumes. He was evaluated by William Rea, M.D., and associates in the ecologic unit of Brookhaven Hospital, in Dallas, Texas, in 1979.

This man's case is of special interest because he was shown to be allergic to only three foods, and they did not cause his arthritis. Before entering the ecology unit he was bedridden for twelve weeks because of his joint sensitivity to reactive chemical agents employed in agricultural and/or food industry chemical technology that contaminated his food.

Arthritis began at age fifty-five with generalized stiffness, pain, and swelling of his fingers, feet, and ankles, and pain in his knees and elbows. He had been on a number of medications, including the steroid prednisone, when he went to the Mayo Clinic in December, 1978. There he was told that he had arthritis in every joint in his body except his back. The steroid was immediately discontinued, and he was started on twelve to fifteen aspirin tablets daily along with physical therapy and heat treatments.

For about six months before going to Mayo, Voors had been very tired at work and was far too tired to engage in any social activities. His hands were so severely involved that the knobs on all the water faucets as well as all the doorknobs in his home were replaced by much larger ones that he could operate with his arthritic hands. From January through March, 1979, he was completely disabled, and during this period when arthritis confined him to bed, he needed assistance in sitting up and getting out of bed. Even though he was on fifteen aspirin a day, he could not walk without help and required assistance boarding and leaving the aircraft that brought him to Dallas.

Mrs. Voors accompanied her husband, and at first she was very much against fasting and told Bill Rea that she was really afraid that her husband who is thin, would starve in the hospital that was supposed to help him. All this changed on the fifth day of fasting on spring water in the controlled environment of the ecology unit. The patient began to feel better; his pain and stiffness were definitely reduced and his weakness was a little less severe despite fasting, which in this arthritic patient was not accompanied by hunger. He was able to sit up and get out of bed without any help, and on the last day of his seven-day fast, Charles Voors walked down the hall unassisted—for the first time in three months!

I am certain that somewhere there is a substantial group of "authorities" on arthritis who will do their very best to convince you that this wonderful, most welcome, and *not unexpected* result—an ecologic triumph—based on unassailable and beautiful logic—of a demonstrated cause-and-effect relationship—is entirely a matter of chance. To them arthritis is a frivolous disease of unknown causation and, for no clearly understood reason, he just happened to have a "spontaneous" remission that just happened to occur while he just happened to be fasting on pure water in a controlled environment.

Mr. Voors continued to improve during his stay in Dr. Rea's ecology unit. Egg, almond, and corn were the only foods that affected him during his postfasting, deliberate, single-food-ingestion challenges, causing acceleration and irregularity of his heart rate, typical changes described by Arthur Coca, M.D., who wrote the *Pulse Test* for the diagnosis of allergies. No foods caused any arthritis symptoms.

After completing a series of ingestion tests with less chemically contaminated, organically produced foods, the foods that did not cause reactions were obtained from regular commercial sources and retested to see if residual agricultural chemicals in his diet—insecticides, fungicides (mold killers) and herbicides (weed killers) and the various chemicals employed in food technology—had an adverse effect on this patient. The chemical substances associated with agrochemical technology were very important in this case; they caused typical flare-ups of his familiar arthritis pains. He also became "stiff all over." In this case foods acted as carriers for the toxic chemicals that caused his arthritis. He also reacted after a brief exposure to the fumes of burning natural gas, for which he was tested in the evening after the personnel in the kitchen had left.

Within an hour he could not use his fingers due to pain and stiffness.

This patient's in-hospital diagnosis and case-management program required five weeks of careful observation and testing. He left the hospital comfortable, his arthritis controlled without the need for medications; and he walked out of the building, took a taxi to the airport, and got on and off the plane without any help. As of mid-August, 1982, he remains well but still is susceptible to the effects of environmental chemicals.

He cannot tolerate a fifteen-minute exposure to the indoor chemical air pollution of a carpet store, freshly painted rooms, or the automotive service garage of his car dealer. The chemical pollutants encountered in these places will cause a moderate to severe flare-up of his familiar joint symptoms, and he becomes very stiff, as in the past—but the symptoms appear from six to eight hours after such exposures have taken place, and he never made the exposure-symptom connection in the past because of the time delay.

Six weeks after returning home from Dr. Rea's ecology unit, this man, who had been totally disabled, was back at his job, working half-days. The college and wedding rings that he had to have made several sizes larger to fit his arthritic fingers have been a source of significant expense to the patient, because to date he has had to have them reduced in size three times to keep them from falling off his steadily improving arthritic fingers. He decided to put the college ring away for a while to keep jewelers' bills down, because his wedding band has to be made smaller again.

Now, 3½ years after his initial ecologic diagnosis and treatment, he continues to follow a rotary-type diet "about 60 percent of the time"; approximately 90 percent of his diet consists of organic foods. If he should eat out twice a day for five days, the cumulative effects of the chemicals in restaurant foods obtained from commercial sources will activate his arthritis.

In his own words: "I think that it is pretty amazing." Mrs. Voors said, "At present he is doing things he couldn't think of doing before—out in the garden—he's even up on the roof."

Mrs. Voors also made another statement that sadly reflects the present state of affairs with respect to the proper treatment of many cases of arthritis. She told me: "Even the people who know him and saw what his arthritis did to him all those years still find it difficult to believe that it [ecologic-allergic diagnosis and treatment] really does help. Some people are so pigheaded!" To that I say "Amen."

Following are some suggestions to aid you as you rid your body of allergy-causing substances.

For Relief of Allergic Symptoms
1. Dr. Randolph's Alkaline Salts.
   a. ⅓ potassium bicarbonate (order 1 pound from your pharmacy)*
   b. ⅔ sodium bicarbonate (baking soda from the grocery)* Take 1 heaping tsp. of this mixture in an 8-ounce glass of spring water, followed with an additional glass of water. May be repeated two or three times in one day. *Not to be used continually for more than* two or three days. (The total single dose is 1 heaping tsp. per 16 oz.)
2. Ascorbic acid or sodium ascorbate (vitamin C). ¼ tsp. (measuring spoon) in 6 to 8 ounces spring water = 1 gram (1000 milligrams). *Repeat every hour if necessary.* If cramping or diarrhea develops, increase interval between each dose to 1½ to 2 hours.
3. Plain sodium bicarbonate (Arm & Hammer baking soda is an excellent and economical form). Take 1 level tsp. in a glass of water and follow immediately with another glass of water. Follow instructions for Dr. Randolph's Alkaline Salts.
4. Alka-Seltzer Gold* (Antacid Formula). 1 tablet in one 8 ounce glass of spring water, to be immediately followed by a second tablet in another 8 ounces of water. Use only Gold in the blue and yellow package, and because it does not contain aspirin. It is very convenient and easy to carry, and it tastes much better than Dr. Randolph's Alkaline Salts. It contains citric acid, which does not bother many patients.
5. Milk of Magnesia—as an Antacid (use only in an unflavored form like Phillip's). 1 to 2 tbsps. Take no water with this. Take 2 to 4 tbsps. as a laxative, in or followed by a glass of spring water.
6. Spring water retention enema. Use 1 quart; may be repeated if necessary. Add 1 tsp. vitamin C and 1 tsp. alkaline salts or 2 tsps. sodium bicarbonate to a quart of spring water. Try to retain the fluid for ten minutes if possible.
7. Epsom salts—as a laxative. Take 1 tsp. in a tall glass of water.
8. Oxygen. Have your physician order it for you from a hospital

---

*It is convenient to prepare several doses of the alkaline salts at one time. Obtain a 2- to 6-ounce bottle with a snug-fitting top and make sure it is dry. The important factor in this preparation is the ratio of sodium to potassium. The size or type of measuring utensil is of no importance if it is clean and dry. Mix 2 parts sodium bicarbonate (use as a measure 2 tablespoons, 2 bottlecapfuls, or 2 whiskey glasses) with 1 part potassium bicarbonate (1 tablespoon or 1 bottlecapful or 1 whiskey glassful). Use the same measure to place the proper amount of each substance into the dry jar or bottle, and mix well by shaking and turning the container.

supply service, because the drugstore cylinders are very expensive. Use 6 liters for 5 minutes; may be repeated during the day as necessary.* *Do not use continually.*

9. Magnesium Citrate—as a laxative. It has a pleasant flavor and usually does an excellent job. Keep in the refrigerator. Directions are 8 to 10 ounces for adults and 4 to 6 ounces for children six to twelve years old.

10. Fleets Phospho Soda (Unflavored). Take 2 to 4 tsps. on arising, thirty minutes before a meal, or at bedtime. Dilute with water, then follow with another glass of water.

11. Antihistamines—if they are tolerated without excessive drowsiness—may be helpful (Benadryl, Chlortrimeton, Teldrin, Actifed, Dimetane, Dimetapp, etc.).

The following will help you keep a careful record of your fasting experiences. Watch for arthritis flare-ups, flulike symptoms, fatigue, depression, nausea, nervousness, stomach cramps, chest tightness, swelling, restlessness, headache, lightheadedness, and the like. Remember that some reactions take time to develop, so pay attention!

Record all your symptoms. To save space and record more information in the box for symptoms and notes, you may use the code on page 184 (HA for headache, JJ for joint pain, MM for muscle pain, F for fatigue, DZ for dizziness, etc.).

---

*Only order oxygen if you have found that it helped you obtain relief that the other simple and economical measures did not provide.

Record of Fasting Reactions or Responses to Foods

Before Fast or Diet		Day 1	Pulse*	Day 2	Pulse	
Clear home of chemicals and fumes	AM Oral Temp.†					
Turn off gas	Weight AM (before breakfast)					
Board plants						
Board pets						
Gather old games and books	PM (at bedtime)					When to take pulse ↔
Stock all necessary supplies, including medications for relief	**Breakfast** Food					Before eating
Make spring-water ice cubes						15 minutes after eating
Have checkup with your personal physician	Reactions, observations, ideas and notes (new symptoms, improvement or worsening of familiar chronic symptoms)					30 minutes after eating
						45 minutes after eating
	Lunch Food					Before eating
						15 minutes after eating
	Reactions, observations, ideas and notes (new symptoms, improvement or worsening of familiar chronic symptoms)					30 minutes after eating
						45 minutes after eating

Before Fast or Diet

	Day 1	Pulse*	Day 2	Pulse	When to take pulse ↕
Supper — Food					Before eating
					15 minutes after eating
					30 minutes after eating
					45 minutes after eating
Reactions, observations, ideas and notes (new symptoms, improvement or worsening of familiar chronic symptoms)					

	Day 3	Pulse	Day 4	Pulse	Day 5	Pulse	When to take pulse ↕
AM Oral Temp.†							
Weight AM (before breakfast)							
PM (at bedtime)							
Breakfast — Food							Before eating
							15 minutes after eating
							30 minutes after eating
							45 minutes after eating
Reactions, observations, ideas and notes (new symptoms, improvement or worsening of familiar chronic symptoms)							

		Day 3	Pulse	Day 4	Pulse	Day 5	Pulse	
Lunch	Food							Before eating
								15 minutes after eating
								30 minutes after eating
								45 minutes after eating
	Reactions, observations, ideas and notes (new symptoms, improvement or worsening of familiar chronic symptoms)							
Supper	Food							Before eating
								15 minutes after eating
								30 minutes after eating
								45 minutes after eating
	Reactions, observations, ideas and notes (new symptoms, improvement or worsening of familiar chronic symptoms)							

*Take your pulse rate after sitting quietly for 5 minutes. Record your pulse just before each test meal and 15, 30, and 45 minutes after eating, or three times a day while fasting.

†Shake the thermometer down to 96° immediately after use. Take your temperature for five minutes as soon as you wake up, before getting out of bed. If you are fasting, take your first pulse of the day as you are taking your temperature. If your resting morning temperature is 97.4 or less, speak to your doctor about the possibility of your having a hypoactive (underactive) thyroid gland that could be responsible for some symptoms. You may learn more about this subject from a book by Dr. Broda Barnes, *Hypothyroidism*, published by T. Y. Crowell, now Harper & Row.

Rinkel Rotary Diversified Diet—Food Elimination Diet

If you do not wish to fast or if for health reasons you are unable to undergo a fast, this rotary elimination diet of less frequently eaten foods can be very effective if you follow the instructions carefully. For example, Dr. Harris Hosen relieved the symptoms of a forty-four-year-old woman who had suffered from arthritis for fifteen years by placing her on a diet of "foods never or infrequently eaten" for six days.

In my office, when testing has been completed, I prescribe patient-specific individual elimination diets with rotation of a combination of test-negative and "uncommon" foods for most of my patients, with considerable success. The diet is a beautiful method of diagnosis that relates foods and symptoms, but it cannot work or be completely effective if chemicals and airborne allergens are ignored and permitted to continue their effects with undiminished intensity.

The food-elimination rotation system is, naturally, a little more complicated than the spring-water fast, but some of you may prefer it since it does allow you to continue eating while still preparing your body for the next part of the diagnostic phase of your arthritis-relief process. For many readers, a diet of infrequently eaten foods will do very well if they are not eaten more often than once every four to seven days. Four days is the minimal spacing; five days or more are better.

To construct this diet, consult the Food Family tables beginning on page 157 and select a group of foods that are uncommon to your diet, and eat only those, on a rotating basis, for five to seven days. You may select *any* foods from the special lists of unrelated plant and animal foods beginning on page 164, and then carefully go over the foods in the classification of plant and animal foods that begins on page 156. Make any choice that you like *except* for those that are part of your usual diet. If you normally consume a lot of goat, venison, or rabbit, for instance, avoid them now even if to everyone else these foods are regarded as exotic.

You may *not* eat any of the foods in the list of major offenders that follows. These are the most common food allergens and may well cause symptoms at the time that we are trying our best to eliminate them. For the present, food mixtures are not permitted because many important foods are hidden in mixtures, such as sugar in catsup and cold cereals and corn in sweeteners and vegetable starch. Milk and soy are in proteins.

Follow these instructions *to the letter*. You may *not* eat any of the following in any form:

    milk
    potato
    beef
    coffee, tea
    corn
    wheat
    orange
    egg
    chicken
    chocolate
    apple
    banana
    carrots
    onion
    tomato
    lettuce
    soy
    sugar
    pork
    peanuts
    string (green) beans
    yeast
    soda
    tap water (unless boiled for 10 minutes or allowed to stand for 3
        days in an open container)

or any food checked as a suspect, for whatever reason, on your personal diet survey in Chapter 6.

The forbidden foods are frequently eaten in some form by most people, and because of your probable heavy exposure to all or most of them, they are highly likely to be the cause of allergic reactions. They must be avoided to eliminate the most common food allergens from your system unless you positively do not eat some of them and you have carefully studied the mixed foods in your diet and know they have not been frequently ingested. Read those labels!

You may choose from among any food on the following lists of plants and animals, except for a food you eat frequently or to which you know you have any kind of reaction. The foods are grouped by families to facilitate your menu planning. The horizontal lines separate the families, and the broken lines and brackets encompass the very closely related foods that must be treated as if they contained the same allergens.

Biologic Classification of Foods

The construction of special, individualized (patient-specific) rotary diversified diets is presently based on the biologic (structural and immunologic) relationship of various foods to each other. We are, however, looking forward to the development of a biochemical classification of foods in the future. To a great extent, I have based this revised biologic classification of foods on the meticulous research of a distinguished and generous friend, Alsoph H. Corwin, Ph.D.,* to whom all of us are indebted. As you progress through your Lifetime Arthritis Relief program, you will return again and again to the fruit of the scholarly research of this dedicated scientist.

After careful study of Dr. Corwin's revised classification of foods, I realized that my fellow ecologists and I had not fully appreciated the clinical value of the Corwin Taxonomic lists of the plant and animal kingdoms. Unfortunately, we were unaware of the fact that *many foods we believed to be related members of the same biologic family actually belonged to different families* that were in the same botanic or zoologic class. For example, lobster, shrimp, and crab belong to different families in the crustacean class, and we incorrectly placed them in a nonexistent "crustacean family" and unnecessarily restricted the frequency of their use in diagnostic and therapeutic diets. We treated these foods as if they were much more closely related than they really are. Use of Dr. Corwin's excellent method of classification gives physicians and patients alike far greater versatility in the formulation of special diets. Unnecessary restrictions in diet planning have been eliminated.

On the other hand, Dr. Corwin has shown that many very closely related species of foods like wheat, rye, and barley (cereal grains in the grass family); casaba, honeydew, and canteloupe (gourd family); or cabbage, brussels sprouts, and broccoli (mustard family) must be considered to be almost identical for allergic individuals until proven otherwise. Therefore, there are certain members within some food

---

*Professor Emeritus of Chemistry, The Johns Hopkins University; Recipients of the Jonathan Forman Gold Medal for meritorious service to humanity through his contributions to Clinical Ecology.

families that should be eaten at least four days apart in rotary diets, because the Rotary Diversified Diet was designed to prevent the reactions that could be caused by allergic overloading. Eating very closely related foods every other day can easily overload a highly allergic person's body with a particular food component that is present in each of the very closely related members of a given food family. In many instances we unknowingly were responsible for allergic overloading because we were not aware of the allergic identity of the foods that we employed at forty-eight-hour intervals, when ninety-six-hour spacing was required.

Food Families—Fish and Animal—Biologically Related Groups

(Horizontal Lines Separate Different Family Groups from Each Other. Brackets and Broken Lines Enclose Allergically Identical Foods.)

sea scallop[1]	lobster	menhaden
bay scallop	American edible	shad
	European edible	
oyster	crayfish	anchovy
clam		salmon (caviar)
butter	crab	Atlantic
geoduck	European edible	caho
pismo	dungeness	dog
quahog	blue	king
soft shell		pink
mussel	honeybee (honey)[2]	sockeye
		trout
abalone	shark	brook
green		brown
pink	beluga	lake
red	sturgeon (caviar)	rainbow
	North American	
edible snail	paddlefish	lake whitefish
North American squid	tarpon	common smelt
octopus	herring	muskellunge
	Atlantic	northern pike
shrimp	Pacific	pickerel
brown grooved	sardine[3]	
pink grooved		
prawn		

1. Imitation sea scallops may be cut from shark or ray with a cookie-cutterlike utensil. Imitation scallops may be served in some restaurants.

2. Honey contains some bee substance and comes from various flowers.

3. Sardines are small or half-grown herrings.

4. Cod and haddock look and taste alike and cost the same; at times one may be substituted for the other in your local fish market. Scrod is young cod.

bigmouth buffalo
black buffalo
sucker

carp
chub

catfish
yellow bullhead

eel
  common
  European
  North American

conger eel

Atlantic cod (scrod)[4]
cusk
haddock
pollack
silver hake
tomcod

mullet
  gray
  striped
  silver
silversides
white bait

barracuda

bass
  Black Sea
  Oriental spotted
  striped
brown grouper
red grouper
red hind
rockfish
speckled hind
white perch

red snapper

grunt
  gray
  common
  yellow

bass (black)
  largemouth
    (bigmouth)
  smallmouth
  spotted
bluegill
longear sunfish
pumpkinseed

pike
yellow perch
walleye

tilefish

bluefish

amberjack
jack mackerel
pompano

dolphin fish

Atlantic croaker
freshwater drumfish
king whiting
silver perch
weakfish

porgy (scup)

albacore
Atlantic bonito
bluefish tuna
Chile bonito
mackerel
  Atlantic
  frigate
  king
  Spanish
skipjack tuna

marlin
sailfish

swordfish

butterfish
harvestfish

dab
flounder

halibut

sole
turbot

ocean perch
rosefish

sea robin
sea tag

puffer

American edible
  bullfrog
European edible
  bullfrog

snapping turtle

diamondback terrapin
green turtle

eastern diamondback
  rattler
western diamondback
  rattler

American alligator

mallard duck
  egg
greylag goose
  egg

partridge (ruffed
  grouse)
prairie chicken

peacock
  egg

domestic chicken
  cornish hen
  egg
  liver
domestic pheasant
Indian pheasant
peafowl
quail

domestic duck
  egg
domestic goose
  egg

guinea fowl

turkey
  egg

dove
pigeon (squab)

opossum

Belgian hare
domestic rabbit
eastern cottontail
jackrabbit
snowshoe rabbit
western cottontail

domestic guinea pig

prairie dog
squirrel
  fox
  gray
  red
woodchuck

beaver

whale

porpoise

dolphin

wolf

bear
  black
  brown
  grizzly
  polar

raccoon

lion
tiger

walrus

sea lion

common seal

elephant

horse

pig (pork)
  bacon
  gelatin
  ham
  lard

hippopotamus

camel
llama

⎰ American elk
⎱ European red deer
- - - - - - - - - - - -
⎧ caribou
⎪ moose
⎨ reindeer
⎩ white-tailed deer
- - - - - - - - - - - -
giraffe

antelope

African buffalo
American bison
brahman
domestic cattle (beef)
  butter
  cheese
  cow's milk
  gelatin
  liver
  other organs
  veal
goat
  cheese
  goat's milk
sheep
  lamb
  mutton

Food Families—Plants—Biologically Related Groups

agar[1]
molds in cheese[2]
mushroom
truffle
yeast
 baker's
 brewer's

Florida arrowroot
 (zamia)

honey[3]

Grass/Grains

bamboo shoots

barley
 malt
 maltose
rye
wheat
 bran
 bulgur
 farina
 flour
  gluten
  graham
  patent
  semolina
  whole wheat
 wheat germ—oil
triticale

oats
 oatmeal

rice
 flour

wild rice

millet
sugar cane
 molasses
 raw sugar
sorghum
 grain
 syrup
corn
 hominy grits
 corn oil
 cornmeal
 corn sugar/sweet-
  ener—syrup
  dextrose (glucose)
 cornstarch
 popcorn
 vitamin C[4]

Chinese water chestnut

Palm

coconut
 oil
 meal
sago palm
 starch (vitamin C)[4]
date palm
 dates
 sugar
palm cabbage

taro
poi
malanga (Arrowroot)

pineapple

Lily

aloe
asparagus
chives
garlic
leek
onion
ramp
shallot
yucca

Fiji arrowroot (tacca)

sarsaparilla

yam
 American
 Chinese
 Indian
 tropical
name

banana
plantain
arrowroot (musa)

saffron
orris root

ginger
turmeric
cardamom

1. Agar has been used in laxatives.
2. Antibiotics are a mold product.
3. Honey comes from different species of flowers.
4. Vitamin C is manufactured from corn. A small number of corn-sensitive individuals do not tolerate this form of vitamin C, and the sago palm product (Nutricology Laboratory) is an excellent source of this nutrient. Another source of vitamin C is prepared from potato. Vitamin C is also manufactured from grape sugar in Europe. Europe.

East Indian arrowroot
  (curcuma)

West Indian arrowroot
  (maranta)

vanilla

black pepper (white)[5]

hickory
pecan
walnut
  black
  English
  white (butternut)

filbert
hazelnut
oil of birch

beechnut
chestnut

breadfruit
fig
hop
mulberry

macadamia nut

buckwheat
garden sorrel
rhubarb

beet[6]
sugar beet (beet sugar)
Swiss chard
- - - - - - - - - - - - - - - -
lamb's quarters
spinach
tampala

olive
  green
  olive oil
  ripe

American pawpaw
custard apple

nutmeg
mace

avocado
bay leaf
cinnamon
sassafras (file)

Chinese lotus

poppy seed

Mustard

broccoli[6]
brussels sprouts
cabbage
cauliflower
celery cabbage
collards
kale
kohlrabi
- - - - - - - - - - - - - - - -
Chinese cabbage
horseradish
mustard
  greens
  seed
radish
rutabaga
turnip
watercress

caper

pomegranate

Brazil nut

Berry[7]

blackberry
boysenberry
dewberry
loganberry
youngberry
raspberry (black, red)
rose hips
strawberry
wineberry

Apple[7]

apple
  butter
  cider
  pectin
  vinegar
crabapple
loquat
pear
quince

Plum[7]

almond
apricot
cherry
peach
  nectarine
plum
  prune

currant
gooseberry

5. Peppercorns have black skins. Whole ground pepper is black. If the skins are removed first, white pepper results.

6. These foods are very closely related and may be tolerated on alternate days by some individuals, but for others they must be considered to be identical in the allergic sense.

7. The rose family has three major divisions—the berry, apple and plum groups. These groups differ enough from each other to be considered as separate families in constructing individual diets.

Legumes

alfalfa
bean[6]
- bush
- garbanzo
- jack
- kidney
- navy
- pinto
- string

bean[6]
- broad
- tonka
- windsor

carob
clover
coumarin
cowpea
fenugreek
flaxseed
gum acacia
gum tragacanth
lentil
licorice
lima bean
mung (sprout)
pea (sweet/green)

pea[6]
- black-eyed
- chick
- split

peanut
pigeon pea
soybean
- flour
- grits
- lecithin
- milk
- oil
- tofu
tamarind

Citrus

angostura
citron
grapefruit
kumquat
lemon
lime
mandarin orange
  tangerine
orange

Barbados cherry
  (acerola)

cassava (meal)
tapioca (Brazilian
  arrowroot)
yucca

litchi nut (lychee)

cashew
mango
pistachio

sugar maple
  maple sugar
  maple syrup

grape
  cream of tartar
  muscadine
  raisin
  slip-skin
  vinegar (wine)
  wine (brandy, cham-
    pagne)

cocoa
  chocolate
cola nut

cottonseed
  meal
  oil
okra

kiwi berry (Chinese
  gooseberry)

tea

passion fruit

papaya

allspice
clove
eucalyptus
guava

arrowroot

Carrot

angelica
anise
caraway
carrot
celeriac
celery
chervil
coriander
cumin
dill
fennel
parsley
parsnip

ginseng
  American
  Asian

Heath

bearberry
blueberry
cranberry
huckleberry
wintergreen

persimmon
  American
  Oriental

chicle

Potato

eggplant
ground cherry
pepper[6]
  garden (green/bell/
    sweet)
  cayenne
  chili
  paprika
  pimento
potato (white/Irish)[4]
tomato
tobacco

Mint

apple mint
basil
bergamot
chia seed
clary
Chinese artichoke
horehound
horse mint
hyssop
lavender
lemon balm
marjoram
oregano
pennyroyal
peppermint
rosemary
sage
savory
spearmint
thyme
water mint

sweet potato

comfrey

---

sesame
  oil
  seeds
  tahini
  butter

---

coffee

---

elderberry

Gourds

Chinese preserving
melon
cucumber

- - - - - - - - - - - - - - -

melon[6]
  canteloupe
  casaba
  crenshaw
  honeydew
  musk
  Persian
  Spanish

- - - - - - - - - - - - - - -

Indian gherkin

- - - - - - - - - - - - - - -

pumpkin (seeds, meal)[6]
summer squash
  crookneck, yellow
  pattypan
  vegetable spaghetti
  zucchini

- - - - - - - - - - - - - - -

large pumpkin[6]
winter squash
  acorn
  butternut
  hubbard
  turban

- - - - - - - - - - - - - - -

watermelon

Lettuce

absinthe
artichoke
  common
  Jerusalem (flour)
burdock root
cardoon
chamomile
chicory
coltsfoot
colstmary
dandelion
endive
escarole
French endive (witloof
  chicory)
goldenrod
lettuce
romaine
safflower oil
salisfy (oyster plant)
santolina
scolymus (Spanish oys-
  ter)
scozzonera (black sal-
  sify)
southernwood
sunflower
  meal
  oil
  seed
tansy
tarragon
vermouth
wormwood

---

juniper (gin)
pine nut

New Zealand spinach

---

cactus pear (prickly)

To make diet planning easier for you, each of the foods in the two following special lists of plant and animal foods is a member of completely different—in the allergic sense—food families. They are unrelated to any other foods you may choose from this food list and may be eaten once in each rotation (5 to 7-plus days) of your Rotary Diversified Diet without looking up the food family to which each of these foods belongs.* However, you can only eat one kind of persimmon, scallop, abalone, clam, bear, rabbit, and so on.

Special Food List: Plant Kingdom Foods in Different Families

Fruits
American pawpaw
Barbados cherry (acerola)
elderberry
grape/raisin
kiwi berry (Chinese gooseberry)
papaya
passion fruit
persimmon
pineapple
pomegranate
prickly pear

Nuts/Seeds
American chestnut
Brazil nut
filbert
litchi nut (Lychee)
macadamia nut
pine nut (pinyon)
poppy seed

sesame seed (tahini)
  tahini paste (raw)
  butter (toasted)

Vegetables
arrowroot—Fiji
arrowroot—Florida (zamia)
arrowroot—maranta starch
arrowroot—Queensland
Chinese water chestnut
Chinese lotus
maté
New Zealand spinach
olive
sweet potato
yam

Spices/Flavors
caper
coffee
comfrey

*This does not mean that there is absolutely no fundamental relationship between any of these foods, even though every one of them does belong to a different biologic family. This is because there are certain natural chemical compounds that look and taste different and come from different plants and animals. Substance X may be present in 20% of the foods you eat and substances Y and Z may be in 50% and 75% respectively. Several colleagues and I are researching such chemicals at this time. Professor Robert W. Gardner, Ph.D., at Brigham Young University in Provo, Utah, originated this work on what he refers to as phenyl food compounds (PFC). To date he and Joseph J. McGovern, Jr., M.D., of Oakland, California, have made some very interesting observations and have indicated that their preliminary use of these multiple-source food-chemical compounds (PFC) shows considerable promise.

flaxseed
maple sugar
sarsaparilla

tea
vanilla

Animal Kingdom Foods in Different Families

Seafood

bay/sea scallops
clam
cockle
oyster
abalone
edible snail
North American squid
crab
lobster
shrimp

dolphin fish
grunt
lake whitefish
North American eel
North American paddlefish
ocean perch
porgy
puffer
red snapper
shark
sole
swordfish
tarpon
tilefish

Insects

honey (bee and flowers)

Amphibians and Reptiles

bullfrog
green turtle
snapping turtle
diamondback terrapin
rattlesnake
American alligator

Meat

antelope
bear
beaver
dolphin
elephant
hippopotamus
horse
llama
opossum
pig
porpoise
rabbit
raccoon
sea lion
seal
walrus

Poultry

guinea fowl
turkey

Fish

anchovy
bluefish
carp
common smelt
conger eel

You may not ingest any substance without very carefully checking the food classifications, special lists, and your replies to the various food related questions, if your elimination diet is to serve its purpose. There's no point in going through this period of single-food testing to help your arthritis if you sabotage yourself by carelessness or poor planning, is there? That means:

> No smoking or exposure to odorous household chemicals or cosmetics.
> No water other than bottled spring water.
> No toothpaste, mouthwash, or regular forms of vitamins (see note 4 on page 160).
> No seasoning (herbs, spices, catsup, mustard, sauces) other than kosher salt, sea salt, lemon,* or any food on the okay list.
> No sweetener other than those on okay list.*

You will eat a different food for each meal, and you will have three single-food meals per day, with "booster" doses of certain foods when indicated. You may eat as much of that food as you wish, but do not overeat.

Spend about fifteen to twenty minutes at each meal, eating slowly for optimum satisfaction. If no symptoms appear within one hour, a "booster" feeding of a quarter to a third of a regular portion of that food is then eaten. Each meal should be separated from the next test meal by at least four hours to allow enough time for reactions to develop—and to clear up spontaneously. If a food causes symptoms, you must postpone the next meal until your symptoms clear up or have become *very* mild. Severe reactions that make you very uncomfortable should be treated by the measures described on pages 149–150.

Foods from the same family should be separated from each other by at least one full day, eaten on the first and third, second and fourth, or third and fifth days of your five-day rotation cycle—forty-eight hours apart. Refer to the food-family lists and you will see, for instance, that you would not eat kohlrabi and rutabaga (or carrot and celery, or artichoke and lettuce) on consecutive days because they belong to the mustard, carrot, and lettuce families, respectively, and must be separated from each other in your diet by a forty-eight-hour period. One of these foods could be eaten on Monday (Day 1) and the other member of the same family may be eaten on Wednesday (Day 3) or Thursday (Day 4). Squash may be eaten on Tuesday (Day 2) and a melon on Thursday (Day 4) or Friday (Day 5). And on Wednesday

---

*Lemon and each sweetener may be used only once during a five- to seven-day rotation cycle.

(Day 3) you could eat potato or kidney beans or beets, and on Friday (Day 5)—forty-eight hours later—you may have either tomato (or eggplant or green pepper), lentils (or lima beans or peanuts), or spinach.

In order for you really to understand how a rotary diversified diet (RDD) is constructed, and to make you feel confident in formulating any future diets, I would like you to go back to pages 157–163 and study the family relationships of the aforementioned foods and any other foods in which you may have an interest. It will not take very long for you to be perfectly comfortable as you become more involved in your diet-planning activities. I want you to understand the full implications of the last two sentences in the previous paragraph, because you can learn a great deal from doing so.

You will note that I suggested you eat squash, a member of the gourd family, on Tuesday, which is Day 2 of the first five-day rotation cycle (I). And I also suggested that you eat an unspecified melon on either Thursday (Day 4) or Friday (Day 5). The spacing between members of the same (gourd) family is forty-eight hours on a Tuesday (Day 2)–Thursday (Day 4) plan, and it is seventy-two hours on the Tuesday (Day 2)–Friday (Day 5) schedule. The minimum forty-eight-hour interval that is required between members of the same family will be preserved between the ingestion of the melon on either Day 4 (Thursday) or Day 5 (Friday) and squash on the following Sunday, which is the second day of Cycle II in this five-day diet. The Thursday–Sunday interval is seventy-two hours, and the Friday–Sunday spacing is forty-eight hours—both eating schedules provide the required minimum time.

Any melon would be a satisfactory selection when eaten forty-eight hours after squash, because squash is sufficiently different from the allergically identical melons and watermelon for this alternate-day exposure to be tolerated. Watermelon is also sufficiently different from the other melons (often referred to as muskmelons) to be eaten forty-eight hours before or after any other melon, but the melons of the muskmelon group are rotated on a four- to seven-day basis because of their "allergic identity."

Potato can be alternated with other members of the potato-nightshade family, and it is a matter of individual choice if the other food from this family (to be eaten two or three days later) is tomato or eggplant or green/sweet/bell pepper. The same applies to kidney beans and the suggested legumes (lentils, lima beans, and peanuts), since they are sufficiently different from the other members of the legume family. However, there is allergic "identity" in the legume family (just as in the gourd family), and when you look up the legumes in the plant-kingdom classification, you will note that a number of beans, including garbanzo, navy, and string beans, are very closely related to kidney beans and require a four- to seven-day rotation because of their allergic similarity. Beets and spinach belong to the goosefoot family and may be eaten forty-eight hours apart.

The reason I indicated that members of the same family (potato, legume, or goosefoot) could be eaten two or three days later was to emphasize the need for proper spacing of related foods. The reason I said that you could have foods that are members of different food families was to show you that any nonrelated foods may also be eaten on the day in a rotation cycle on which a related food might have been scheduled.

You may eat a given food in any form—raw, cooked, steamed, baked, broiled, solid, pureed, or juiced—and even stir-fried in the near future. Just remember that foods in different forms are still the same food: carrot juice, raw carrots, cooked carrots, and pureed carrots are all carrot and should not be repeated within the next five days.

Use the form on page 169 to plan your menus. You will find a selection of five-day rotary-diet sequences with three or more foods to choose from for each meal on page 170. Any questions you have about the system can be answered by studying those samples and comparing them with the food-family classification charts for plants and animals. After designing your individual diet, please double-check it against the food lists to make sure it follows the guidelines.

Keep careful records of your reactions during the Elimination Diet, using the chart on pages 151–153.

Refer to the previous section on the spring-water fast for further suggestions.

Five-Day Rotary Diet

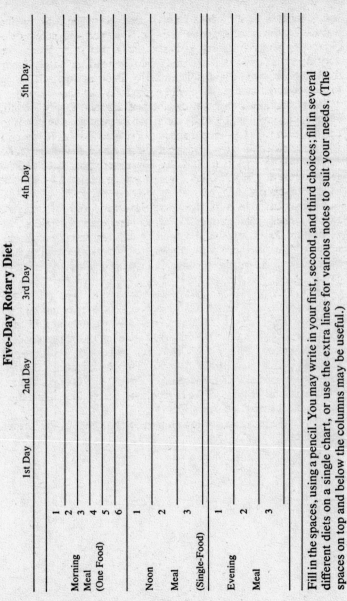

	1st Day	2nd Day	3rd Day	4th Day	5th Day
Morning 1					
Meal 2					
(One Food) 3					
4					
5					
6					
Noon 1					
Meal 2					
(Single-Food) 3					
Evening 1					
Meal 2					
3					

Fill in the spaces, using a pencil. You may write in your first, second, and third choices; fill in several different diets on a single chart, or use the extra lines for various notes to suit your needs. (The spaces on top and below the columns may be useful.)

Rotary Diversified Diet (Food Elimination Diet)

Sample Five-Day Diversified Rotation of Foods—Major Offenders Omitted

Day of Cycle	1	2	3	4	5
Morning Meal	prune (plum)	pineapple (pineapple)	peach (plum)	melon (gourd)	grapefruit (citrus)
	wild rice (grain)	arrowroot	oatmeal (grain)	papaya	buckwheat
	strawberry (berry)	blueberry	persimmon	pear (apple)	currants
Noon Meal	squash (gourd)	string bean or kidney bean (legume)	cauliflower or broccoli (mustard)	parsnip or celery (carrot)	beets (goosefoot)
	rutabaga or turnip (mustard)	red snapper	walnuts (walnuts)	lima bean or lentil (legume)	avocado
		sweet potato (morning glory)	spinach (goosefoot)		chestnuts
Evening Meal	turkey (bird) or flounder or deer/venison	lamb (bovine) or cod or swordfish	sole or rabbit or shrimp	scallops or salmon or duck	tuna or bear or lobster
	and/or dates (palm)	and/or mango (cashew)	and/or macadamia nuts	and/or cashews (cashew)	and/or pecans (walnut)
	(palm)		and/or coconut		

Note: All the foods on this sample diet are compatible with each other if eaten as scheduled and correctly spaced. The food family is listed in parentheses under each food. After Day 5, repeat the cycle. Remember that this is a sample diet for you to study; it cannot possibly be satisfactory for everyone. The most common food offenders like beef, egg, chicken, milk, potato, corn, onion, soy, pork, carrot, peanut, chocolate, cane sugar, tomato and wheat, lettuce, string beans, apple, orange, banana, etc. do not appear on this menu. Select a single food for each test meal; you may choose any food from among the three to five foods listed for each meal.

After you have carefully followed your fast or special diet for five days, you will have removed most if not all of the residues of the previously eaten offending foods from your system. This includes all the arthritis-evoking substances to which you are sensitive and are ill from. If some traces of food do remain in your system, it is very likely that you have reduced their amounts to a level that is below your threshold for developing an allergic reaction. There is an excellent chance that you feel a lot better already, and if you do, I would be happy to receive a letter from you.*

Now you are ready to begin the very important period of self-testing to identify the specific dietary substances you have been eating that cause you to have symptoms. And you are probably in for some exciting and enlightening surprises as your carefully planned and properly followed diet begins to pinpoint the factors that have made you so uncomfortable for so long. In addition, your efforts may help a great deal with many nonarthritic health conditions that you have come to accept as part of your life and can, at last, become free of.

* I would like to know, day by day, what your withdrawal symptoms were, if they were long-term familiar ones, and how you now feel at the end of your fast or special diet. My address is: 3 Brush Street, Norwalk, Connecticut 06850. Print *Arthritis Report* on the lower left of the envelope.

8

The Six-Day Rotary Diagnostic Diet

Now that you have fasted or dieted your body free of all the foods that may have been causing your chronic arthritis, its flare-ups, and perhaps some other unrecognized allergic disorders, you will probably be able to determine which foods they actually are. The series of six-day diet cycles described here will provide you the opportunity you have been waiting for to observe the effects of all the food you've been eating since your arthritis symptoms began. With a little more effort and a little bit of luck, your problem may clear up or be much better very soon.

The rotary (rotation) diet system is derived from the work of Dr. Herbert Rinkel, and the principles on which it is based are both logical and scientifically valid. All foods—plant and animal—technically are classified into biologic groups that include "families" that share certain characteristics. For accurate dietary diagnosis and treatment, you must keep the intake of related foods (from the same family) separated from each other by an interval of at least forty-eight hours—every other day—with a few exceptions.

Before you begin, refresh your memory about how to prepare your individualized six-day diet by referring to the general instructions beginning on page 140 in the previous chapter.

The principle of this Rotary Diagnostic Diet is the same as that of the Food Elimination Diet, but its purpose is different. In this series of rotating menus, you will intentionally introduce foods to which you may be sensitive for diagnostic purposes. Because elimination of probable offenders has removed those substances from your system, your body will now react to them with extra intensity when they are ingested one at a time. You can easily make the cause-and-effect connections between eating specific foods and provoking flare-ups of your arthritis as well as manifestations of any other food-related allergic ailments you may have.

My Lifetime Arthritis Relief system works like this: for six days you will follow a menu composed of eighteen single-food meals, eating three meals a day. You will eat eighteen different foods, one at a time. You will not eat the same food twice during the six-day cycle, and foods from the same plant or animal family will be separated from each other by at least forty-eight hours. You will keep careful and detailed records on the forms provided of what you eat and of *any* reactions that occur after eating. This certainly includes arthritis flare-ups as well as any other food-induced allergic responses you may have. When you have completed the first six-day cycle, you will study your records to decide what you should do during the second and third cycles of the Rotary Diagnostic Diet series. You can retest any foods that you wish to for whatever reason.

You will probably eliminate foods to which you had a particularly unpleasant reaction, but you may repeat such offenders if you wish to confirm this finding—or perhaps show your doctor what a food can do to you. You may add new foods to your rotary diet to replace major offenders, and you should carefully observe and record the effects of the newly added foods. I hope that you made your home as chemical-, dust-, pet-, and mold-free as possible before starting the food tests. It would be a shame to put in this much effort and perhaps significantly interfere with the diagnostic accuracy of the results of food testing because of confusing and avoidable symptoms from other sources that you could have eliminated. Please do your very best to do it right—so much depends on controlling as many factors as possible at the same time.

Instructions for Cycle I

Select your foods. Refer to the list of common food offenders and your personal diet surveys in Chapter 6 and select a group of eighteen foods to start with. Your newly acquired knowledge of food allergy and food addiction will make the choices easy for you, because the probable offenders are waving red flags at you. By eating those prime suspects in individual, well-separated, single-food-ingestion tests, you are probably going to experience some dramatic evidence of the relationship of some foods to your arthritis. And you will learn how important food allergy really is.

This is a very sensitive, highly accurate, biologically sound method of diagnosing and treating food allergies. The more you use it, the more you will come to appreciate its clinical value and the beautiful logic that it is based on. If you cannot find eighteen foods on your personal diet survey list, add some from the list on page 155, since these commonly eaten foods are most likely to cause significant reactions in many people. Wheat, beef, egg, soy, and corn are very often found to be major troublemakers and should be tested if you eat them twice a week.

Organize your menus. Categorize each of the foods you have selected according to their food families by referring to the classification of plant and animal foods that begins on page 157.

Now, using the blank form on page 176, *plan and chart your meals* the first few times, using a pencil with a good eraser. Remember:

> You will eat one food per meal (single-food meals).
> You will eat only three meals a day*
> Foods from the same family must be separated by at least forty-eight hours.

Some allergic individuals cannot tolerate a forty-eight hour spacing for members of the grass (grain) group, because they are more closely related to each other than the other foods. For some people the spacing must be four days or even greater; a cereal could only be eaten once in this six-day cycle. Wheat, corn, or rice could be eaten on Day 2 every six days or wheat could be eaten during the first cycle, corn during the second, and rice on Day 2 of the third cycle of rotation. The rotation system is very flexible in some ways and you can follow two different rotation cycles at once by eating wheat, corn, and barley on a four-day rotation with each other while keeping "isolated" some foods for testing that may be a little difficult to plan.

Test wheat with matzo, dry puffed wheat, shredded wheat, Ralston, Wheatena, or spaghetti boiled in spring water. You

---

*The second evening meal (snack) is not eaten in the early diagnostic phase of your diet, the point we are at now.

Your Individualized 6-Day Rotary Diversified Diet (RDD)*

This form can be used for both planning and abbreviated record-keeping. When you eat a meal, note how much of the food you ate. Permission is granted for you to photocopy this form for later use, too.

	1st Day	2nd Day	3rd Day	4th Day	5th Day	6th Day
Time:						
Morning Meal						
Reaction	NR_SL_ER_	NR_SL_ER_	NR_SL_ER_	NR_SL_ER_	NR_SL_ER_	NR_SL_ER_
Time:						
Noon Meal						
Reaction	NR_SL_ER_	NR_SL_ER_	NR_SL_ER_	NR_SL_ER_	NR_SL_ER_	NR_SL_ER_
Time:						
Evening Meal						
Reaction	NR_SL_ER_	NR_SL_ER_	NR_SL_ER_	NR_SL_ER_	NR_SL_ER_	NR_SL_ER_

NR = No Reaction   SL = Slight Reaction   ER = Extreme Reaction

A Sample 6-Day Rotary Diet
(With 48-hour spacing between members of the same food family)

These are single foods. Do not combine with other foods, herbs, or spices. This comes later.

	1st Day	2nd Day	3rd Day	4th Day	5th Day	6th Day
Morning Meal	apples	wheat** (Wheatena, shredded wheat, puffed wheat, matzo, or spaghetti) Ⓖ	oranges or fresh juice	corn (grits, meal or popcorn) Ⓖ	eggs (chicken) Ⓟ (poached, soft or hard-boiled) Ⓟ	brown rice† Ⓖ
Noon Meal	tomato Ⓝ	lettuce	white potato Ⓝ	milk Ⓑ	carrots (raw and/or cooked) Ⓟ	sweet potatoes
Evening Meal	chicken Ⓟ	beef Ⓑ	sole	turkey*	haddock	pork

Ⓟ – poultry
Ⓖ – grass family
Ⓑ – bovine family
Ⓝ – nightshade family

*Turkey can be eaten 24 hours before (chicken) egg because they are in different families.

†Some allergic individuals can not tolerate a 48-hour spacing for members of the grass (grain) group, because they are more closely related to each other than the other foods. For some people the spacing must be four days or even greater; a cereal could only be eaten once in this six-day cycle. Wheat, corn, or rice could be eaten on Day 2 every six days or wheat could be eaten during the first cycle, corn during the second, and rice on Day 2 of the third cycle of rotation. Then add banana to Day 4, and pineapple to Day 6. The rotation system is very flexible in some ways and you could follow two different rotation cycles at once by eating wheat, corn, and barley on a four-day rotation with each other while keeping the other foods on six-day spacing.

may eat a combination of these all-wheat products for a single test.

Test baker's yeast by eating a package of it "straight" or dissolved in spring water or a test-negative juice.

Test rye by eating plain (unseasoned) rye crackers or pure rye cereal.

Test other grains and cereals by boiling them in spring water. Some cereal grains belong to different tribes in the same family and some are members of the same tribe. Barley, rye, and wheat are very closely related, and some authorities consider them to be allergically identical and require a four-day interval between them. Some have found that all grains must have four-day spacing for certain individuals. Care is required. Remember, no milk and sugar—only sea salt is permitted as seasoning.

Poach eggs in spring water or eat them semihard or soft-boiled.

Test cane sugar by dissolving two tablespoons in a glass of spring water and drinking the mixture.

Eat Baker's chocolate "straight" or grate two or more 1-ounce squares into spring water or a pure juice that you know you are not sensitive to.

To test spices, herbs, oils, and other common allergens, sprinkle on or cook with proven test-negative foods, one at a time.

Keep detailed records for short-term planning and future reference. The blank menu form on page 176 provides limited space for brief reminder notes on your reactions, but you should keep a diary in your own style. However you do it, you will want to include your prebreakfast and postsupper bedtime weight each day as well as:

> the time and date of each single-food test meal
> the amount of food eaten
> your pulse (heart) rate before and after eating
> the time of your reaction
> the symptoms evoked (arthritic and others)
> the severity of symptoms
> the fact that there was no reaction

Changes in pulse rate (in the absence of other symptoms) indicate the presence of a potential food allergen that would probably cause symptoms if it were to be taken too often or, perhaps, in very large quantities or with alcohol. An increase or decrease of eight to ten or more beats per minute is significant. Take your pulse for a full minute after sitting quietly for five minutes. The pulse rate is to be taken just before test meals and every fifteen to twenty minutes for one hour after the single-food test meal has been eaten. If your pulse is elevated fifteen to twenty minutes after eating, take your first reading at five or ten minutes to detect the earliest change. I have one patient whose pulse accelerated twenty to thirty beats while he was still chewing the test food and it was being absorbed sublingually. There is an interesting paperback on this subject, *The Pulse Test*, by Arthur Coca, M.D., that may be purchased at health food stores and elsewhere.

IMPORTANT NOTE—If you are still having a reaction when it is time for your next test meal, postpone that meal until your reaction clears. By doing this you will avoid having to unravel and retest because of confusing situations involving the possibility that two overlapping reactions may have been taking place at the same time.

If you have a severe reaction to a food, you can relieve it by the techniques listed on pages 149–150. The basic idea is (1) to decrease or stop active symptoms; (2) to prevent additional absorption of the cause of the reaction by removing the still-remaining portion of the offending food from the intestines to eliminate the source of the trouble. Two Alka Seltzer Gold tablets in 16 ounces of spring water (one tablet per 8-ounce glass of water; take 2 glasses), along with a quart-size two-level-teaspoon sodium bicarbonate (baking soda) enema are a good way to start. Remember, these food-test reactions are not "withdrawals." They are allergic flare-ups of chronic conditions that have been converted to acute reactions by a five-day period (or longer) of fasting or rotary diet elimination of the specific food(s) causing your arthritis and/or other allergies.

When you have completed the first six-day cycle of your Diagnosic Rotary Diversified Diet, summarize your reactions on the blank form on page 183. A sample of a complete summary form with a symptom key is on page 184. The idea is to rate the foods that caused no reaction, those causing a slight reaction, and the foods that evoked an important reaction (moderate or severe; brief or prolonged), and the symptoms brought on by the test food.

Instructions for Rotation Cycles II and III

Follow these cycles the same way you followed Rotation Cycle I, with these exceptions.

> In choosing your foods for diagnostic purposes, omit those foods that your records show you had no reaction to in Cycle I: They will be excellent for your future allergy-free diet, since they were tolerated. In an occasional case there may be so many discomfort-causing reactions that the diet may be planned to include some probable nonoffenders in order to give the highly reactive individual some relief from test-evoked symptoms.

The most important foods to test are:

> Those "prime suspects" you could not fit into Cycle I— your personal suspects and untested foods from the common major offenders list.

Any tested foods the reactions to which you are doubtful about. If you got only a vague reaction to some food, try it again; if you reacted to a food eaten in a large quantity, try it again in a smaller portion to see if a smaller amount is tolerated.

Double-check, if you wish, any food that induced a sharp reaction during Cycle I. If the uncomfortable experience is repeated, you will have no doubt about its significance for you. Some feeding-challenge reactions are of such intensity that you may not wish to repeat the experience!

What Have You Learned?

Study your various records and questionnaires carefully. Make a list of those foods that provoked reactions—the ones to which you are sensitive—and arrange them according to their biologic family groups to see what your pattern of reactions turns out to be. These are the illness-causing foods you are going to avoid for the present.

Next, list the foods to which you do not react presently or from which you had only mild symptoms. These are the foods you might be able to eat without restriction for a while, but it is best to rotate carefully the currently innocent nonreaction-causing and mild-reaction-causing foods (minor offending foods) in order not to lose your tolerance to them. It is in your best interest not to lose safe foods. Do not cause unnecessary problems due to additional food restrictions that could have been prevented.

Your reactions to the special diagnostic diet have proved that you are food allergic and that some foods cause the joint and muscle symptoms of your arthritis. More important, you have learned that you should be able to control your food-related allergic arthritis by regulating your diet! By carefully following the diagnostic cycles and studying your reactions and results, you should now have a clear picture of the specific foods in each of the various food families that can cause your arthritis to flare up. You may not react to all foods in a family; test each one before you decide to eliminate any member of a family, or there may be unnecessary self-imposed restrictions in your diet. You have demonstrated to your own satisfaction, in your own arthritic body, what my colleagues and I have proven in our offices and in the hospital-based units in thousands of cases over the course of many years: arthritis is very often caused by food allergy, and this allergic disorder can be cured by removing offending foods from your diet.

You have also seen that your familiar arthritis symptoms can and will return if you reintroduce those same test-identified foods to your diet before you have regained your tolerance to a cyclic offender or if you have not allowed enough time for the cumulative effects of an arthritis-causing food to drop below your reaction threshold level.

You have shown yourself, your family, and your friends that these now-predictable ups and downs are not spontaneous flare-ups or spontaneous remissions, as the conventional rheumatologists and other followers of the Arthritis Foundation point of view would have it. Many remissions and exacerbations of arthritis are controllable allergic reactions that are caused by specific dietary substancs. Once they are identified, these foods can be eliminated or eaten less often (at tolerated intervals), and the disease will cease to be active.

There are many possible arthritis-provoking nonfood factors in your environment—the substances that are present in the air you breathe. Remember, you may have reduced them to a level below your threshold by your environmental cleanup before starting the rotary diets, so you may be sensitive to those substances as well as to the foods you eat.

If you have experienced no dramatic results from your diet, it is especially important that you carefully study the next chapter. If you have improved so much that you have become convinced that a single food or groups of foods is the only cause of your arthritis, the information in the next chapter is still valuable to you.

Clearing up an important food allergy problem often reduces the arthritic person's total allergic stress load to a degree that significantly lessens the impact of natural airborne allergens and atmospheric chemical pollutants—for a while. And then the environmental factors gradually build up and cause trouble to appear again. Furthermore, you and I are concerned with your overall health and well being, as well as with your arthritis. I want you to learn as much as you can about bioecologic physical and mental disorders to be certain you will become as well as possible.

Summary of Food Reactions for Rotary Diversified Diet Preparation

Place the name of each food in the proper column and indicate the symptoms it caused.

See example of completed summary below.

Severe Reaction	Moderate Reaction	Slight Reaction	No Reaction	Foods Not Tested

Example of a Completed Summary of Food Reactions for Your Guidance

Severe Reaction	Moderate Reaction	Slight Reaction	No Reaction
pork HA, V	milk F, Dz	haddock DP, VB	sole
scallops VB, DP	corn I	egg I	lamb
tuna CR, HA	vinegar HA, Dz	rice Dz	coffee
cabbage N	banana BL	grape F, N	white potato
wheat JJ	peach Sn	tea HA	cane sugar
chicken V	string beans N	onion ND	baker's yeast
	beef Dr	tomato I, CH	oats
	peanut HA	turkey CR	broccoli
	pecan I	orange N, HA	salmon
			celery
			lettuce
			apple
			cucumber
			onion
			cola
			liver

Symptom Key
DP—depressed
ND—nasal discharge
CH—cough
MM—muscle pain

HA—headache
VB—visual blurring
CR—cramps

N—nausea
JJ—joint pain
V—vomiting

F—fatigue
Dz—dizziness
I—itching

Bl—bloated
Dr—diarrhea
Sn—sneezing

9

How to Identify and Control the Environmental Causes of Your Arthritis

A woman who read *Dr. Mandell's Five-Day Allergy Relief System* wrote to say she was positive that she had ruled out the possibility of food allergy. Although she had fasted on spring water and followed a single-food diagnostic rotary diet religiously, these measures had no beneficial effect on her symptoms, which persisted throughout her fast. On investigation I found she had learned very little from the diet. She had not properly controlled her heavy exposure to the chemical pollutants and inhalant allergens in her home environment, and these factors alone could make her as ill as she could be whether she had food allergy or not.

When my technicians tested her for sensitivities to airborne allergens and chemical agents, her responses indicated that many of her chronic symptoms were undoubtedly allergic reactions triggered by pollens, molds, and environmental chemicals, as she suspected. But we also found that she had many food allergies and could not have improved during fasting because her severe reactions to pollens, molds, and chemical pollutants were enough to keep her very ill by themselves.

This patient is a typical case of broad-based, multiple sensitivities that encompass the three major groups of environmental offenders—foods, chemicals, and natural (native) airborne inhalants.

It is easy to understand why environment has such an important effect on our health. We are surrounded by chemicals that no previous generation of humankind has ever encountered. New technological discoveries have filled the air we breathe with new artificial substances. Chemical laboratories have created the synthetic petrochemical threads of our clothing; the household furnishings; the housekeeping and laundering materials we handle each day; hair spray, air freshener, deodorant, disinfectant, cologne, aftershave lotion, and so on. At one or more stages of the growing and marketing processes, much of the food we eat is exposed to and treated with numerous chemical agents—and some are toxic.

Think for a moment about what that means. Human evolution took millions of years: to achieve even a single minor adaptation, human beings may have to pass through many, many generations before there is a slight altering of man's genetic structure. The countless new chemicals in our environment have simply not been around long enough for our bodies to have developed biologic measures by which we can adapt to them—especially the growing numbers of toxic substances. The body fights some of them off with allergylike protective responses like congestion, swelling, muscle spasm, mucus secretion, sneezing, coughing, vomiting, diarrhea, and the like.

Cockroaches and other insects have a better chance in this new environment than people do. Because those creatures go through many generations in a single year, many of them are able to evolve the necessary protective adaptations. For this reason the manufacturers of insecticides must continually develop stronger new formulas for sprays and powders that will be effective in controlling the new generations of pests that are the offspring of the survivors that were immune to the "old" insecticides. People are not so lucky. As many as half of all allergy sufferers are susceptible to some of the many active chemicals that get into our food and water supplies and pollute the air that we must breathe to exist, polluted or not.

Remember, in the unending process of inhaling life-sustaining oxygen, you may also breathe in the fumes of a noxious air polluting substance to which you are sensitive. Through the lungs it passes into the bloodstream and then to all parts of your body. If you touch it or otherwise come into contact with it, it may pass through the skin and mucous membranes into the circulation, with the same end effect. And if you ingest any food or beverage that has been treated with or contaminated by a chemical to which you are sensitive, both food or beverage and chemicals travel from the digestive system to organs throughout your body via your circulation; without your being aware of your sensitivity, many important parts of your body—internal structures—are being exposed. It is interesting to note, for instance, that while many people who are heavy smokers are addictively allergic to some factors in tobacco smoke, there are many nonsmokers who are acutely sensitive to the chemicals used in the growing and processing of the tobacco leaves and cigarette paper.

A partial list of other commonly encountered agents and products to which many of my patients have been proven to be sensitive will give you some idea of the scope of the problem. These commonly encountered products include insect spray, furniture polish, floor wax, detergent, laundry bleach, gasoline, diesel fuel, car and truck exhaust fumes, roofing tar, blacktop, perfume, hair spray, cosmetics, room deodorizer, shoe polish, cat repellent, waterproofing sprays, turpentine, ammonia, chlorine and fluoride (and therefore drinking water and many toothpastes), natural gas, ink eradicators, felt-tip permanent marking pens, typewriter ribbons, carbon paper, industrial floor cleaning powders, tobacco smoke, exhaust fumes from factories and burning dumps, art supplies, disinfectants, and fuels for heating systems, among others.

Diagnosing Your Chemical Susceptibility and Allergic Sensitivities to Inhalants

As you might imagine, in some instances it is a very simple matter to test yourself for chemical sensitivities. In others it is difficult, because the suspect substances are so pervasive or so well hidden. At the Alan Mandell Center for Bio-Ecologic Diseases, we have often produced typical episodes of arthritis flare-ups in arthritic and otherwise allergic patients whose history indicates the presence of chemical sensitivities. This is easily accomplished by placing one to four drops of a solution prepared from the suspected chemical under the patient's tongue. Of course, you cannot do that at home, but there are ways in which you can determine many of the important environmental substances that trigger your arthritis. And there are ways of reducing the levels of pollutants in your home (and, with employer cooperation, at work) that will benefit not only your arthritis but your total state of health as well as that of your family.

You may already have a general idea of what chemical agents cause you problems. For instance, does your arthritis flare up at one time of year more than at other times? What else happens indoors and outdoors, at home or at work at that time of year? Are fallen leaves and grass clippings undergoing decay by molds? Are trees pollenating, with yellow powder all over? Are you having the house or the trees sprayed? Is traffic near your home heavier than usual? Are you putting clothing away in mothballs? Taking clothing out of them? Are windows shut tight, trapping heating and cooking gas, cigarette smoke, or other pollutants inside? Do you have a marathon spring cleaning with many cleaning agents? Are you painting? Has the exterminator come? Are you spraying your garden? Do you swim in a chlorinated pool? Are you burning fires frequently in the fireplace? Is there any special chemical exposure going on at work, school, or place of recreation? These are chemical and inhalant exposures that are among the many causes of "seasonal" arthritis.

Keep asking questions; keep looking. Does your arthritis bother you more in one place than in others? In several places? Why? What goes on in the places that affect you? What do they use? What did they do that bothered you before you got there? Are you affected at work more than at home, for instance, or vice versa? Indoors or outdoors? In the car, commuting on a highway? When you return to the city from a country vacation? When the lawn is cut? Out in a meadow? During hay-fever seasons? When the pollen count is reported along with the daily news? When you visit a country cottage surrounded by pine trees? Think about the chemical and biologic differences among your different environments.

To get a better idea of whether you are allergic to environmental chemicals, please complete the following questionnaire.

Chemical and Inhalant Questionnaire A

In addition to or separately from allergies to food, you may be sensitive to many of the potential offending substances that are often encountered in the environments of your daily activities. For instance:

Do you experience an arthritis flare-up or any other symptoms under any of the following conditions:

	Yes	No
During prolonged periods of damp weather?	___	___
When you smell mildew?	___	___

When you are near hay or straw (as at the circus, in a barn, near a haystack, on a hay ride)? When

Yes No

you go into an old, damp, musty house, a damp
basement, a shed or cellar? When you enter a
closet in which are stored old shoes, ice skates,
ski boots, unused luggage, gloves or other leather
goods? If you eat cheese (especially the types
with visible mold) mushrooms, cantaloupe,
vinegar (pickles, catsup, mustard, mayonnaise,
salad dressing) or sauerkraut, or drink buttermilk
or other fermented beverages (beer, wine,
whiskey)? When you sit in musty old overstuffed
furniture?   ___ ___

When you are near dry leaves or a compost pile? ___ ___

Are you better off when the snow has been on the
ground for several days?   ___ ___

A *yes* to any of the previous questions indicates that there is
probably an allergy to molds or yeast.

Do you experience a flare-up:

Yes No

When the house is being cleaned or swept?   ___ ___

When using the vacuum cleaner?   ___ ___

When emptying the vacuum cleaner or carpet
sweeper?   ___ ___

When the rugs are being beaten?   ___ ___

When the bed is being made or the mattress turned? ___ ___

During spring housecleaning?   ___ ___

When the first cold snap of autumn comes and heat
is turned on?   ___ ___

In such places as theaters, churches, grocery
stores, department stores, libraries, or areas in
your home like the attic, basement or your
bedroom where dust is noted?   ___ ___

A *yes* to any of the previous questions indicates a probable allergy
to house dust.

Do you experience a flare-up:

	Yes	No
When lying on a feather pillow?	___	___
When fluffing pillows?	___	___
When using a down comforter?	___	___
When you are near chickens, ducks, geese, pigeons, parrots, turkeys, canaries or other birds?	___	___
When you are around anyone who works with poultry or other fowl?	___	___

A *yes* to any of the previous questions may indicate an allergy to feathers.

Do you experience a flare-up:

	Yes	No
When you are around any of the following animals: dogs, cats, horses, goats, rabbits, cows, hogs, sheep?	___	___
When you handle or come into contact with any of the following: furs, rugs, certain articles of clothing, dress goods, blankets, gloves, hats, toy animals or brushes?	___	___

A *yes* to any of the above questions indicates a likely allergy to animal hairs, dander and odors, or house dust or synthetic fibers.

Do you experience a flare-up:

	Yes	No
When using scented face, talcum, body, bath or tooth powder?	___	___
In beauty salons or barber shops?	___	___
When you are around people who use a lot of powder or perfume?	___	___

A *yes* to any of the previous questions indicates a probable "chemical" allergy to petroleum-derived chemicals or the orris root present in some cosmetics.

Do you experience a flare-up:

	Yes	No
When you handle or are around animal or poultry feed?	___	___
When you use certain hair-wave sets, shampoos or tonics?	___	___

A *yes* to any of the previous questions indicates an allergy to cottonseed and/or flaxseed.

Do you experience a flare-up:

	Yes	No
When you smoke?	___	___
When you are around those who are smoking, especially in small rooms or cars?	___	___
When in nightclubs or other smoky places?	___	___
When you are in rooms where there is residual room odor from ashtrays or on another person's clothing, hair, or breath?	___	___

A *yes* to any of the previous questions indicates a probable chemical allergy to tobacco smoke or the chemicals used in tobacco processing.

Do you experience a flare-up:

	Yes	No
When you are exposed to household insect powder or sprays?	___	___
When you are exposed to powders, sprays or crystals used for mothproofing purposes?	___	___
When you are exposed to dusting powders, liquids or sprays used in the home or garden or on the lawn or trees?	___	___
When an exterminator has been at your home or office?	___	___

A *yes* to any of the previous questions indicates a likelihood of allergy to pyrethrum, derris root, paradichlorobenzene, or highly toxic sprays.

Please glance back over your answers. If you are chemically sensitive, you probably have more *yes* answers in some sections than in others. That pattern will give you a general idea of which types of environmental substances may be linked to your arthritis symptoms.

The following questionnaires will allow you to become more specific.

Chemical Questionnaire B

Just as you reviewed food exposures and reactions in your personal diet survey, you will now look for chemical clues in the same way. Some allergists and all bioecologists have long known that persons who are more sensitive to the odor of a given substance than other people are likely to have an allergylike sensitivity to that substance. Similarly, odors that you love or find sickening are usually emitted by chemicals that affect you badly. Therefore, please record your responses to the following chemical agents by placing a check mark in the column that applies to you.

If something gives you certain symptoms (makes you sick) or relieves a particular symptom or symptoms, you should indicate this by placing code letters instead of check marks in the column. For example, if natural gas fumes give you a headache, write *HA* in the "Made sick by" column. If gasoline makes you dizzy, write *Dz* in this column. If kerosene, nail polish, or paint thinner relieves a headache, place *HA* in the "Feel good from" column. You may make up your own code to record chemically related symptoms. You might employ some of the following: N—nausea, V—vomiting, Dr—diarrhea, Cr—cramps, F—fatigue, S—sleepy, Nr—nervous, JP—joint pain, MP—muscle pain, R—restless, VB—visual blurring, Bl—bloating, Co—cough, Sn—sneeze, NO—nasal obstruction, and so on.

*Petroleum Products**

COAL, OIL, GAS, and COMBUSTION PRODUCTS

	Love or crave	Dislike or hate	Made sick by	Feel good from	Feel neutral about	Frequent exposure to
massive outdoor exposure to coal smoke						
smoke from coal-burning stoves, furnaces, or fireplaces						
odors of natural gas fields						
odors of escaping utility gas						
odors of burning utility gas						
odors of gasoline						
garage fumes and odors						
automotive or motorboat exhausts						
odor of naphtha, cleaning fluids or lighter fluids						
odor of recently cleaned clothing, upholstery or rugs						
odor of naphtha-containing soaps						
odor of nail polish or nail-polish remover						
odor of brass, metal or shoe polish						

*The first extensive questionnaire of this type was prepared by my dear friend and mentor Theron G. Randolph, M.D., who coined the term *chemical susceptibility* and conducted basic and advanced studies in this extremely important field, which has grown from his basic concepts. Most of this data appears in the current edition of *Clinical Ecology,* edited by L. Dickey (Springfield, Ill.: Charles C. Thomas, 1976).

	Love or crave	Dislike or hate	Made sick by	Feel good from	Feel neutral about	Frequent exposure to
odor of fresh news-papers						
odor of kerosene						
odor of kerosene or fuel-oil lamps or stoves						
odor of kerosene or fuel-oil space heaters or fur-naces						
diesel engine fumes from trains, buses, trucks, or boats						
lubricating greases or crude oil						
fumes from automo-biles burning an excessive amount of oil						
fumes from burning greasy rags						
odors of smudge pots as road markers or frost inhibitors						

MINERAL OIL, PETROLEUM JELLY, WAXES, and COMBUSTION PRODUCTS

	Love or crave	Dislike or hate	Made sick by	Feel good from	Feel neutral abut	Frequent exposure to
mineral oil as con-tained in hand lo-tions and medica-tions						
mineral oil as a laxa-tive						

	Love or crave	Dislike or hate	Made sick by	Feel good from	Feel neutral about	Frequent exposure to
cold cream or face or foundation cream						
petroleum jelly or petroleum-containing ointments						
odors of floor, furniture, or bowling-alley wax						
odors of glass wax or similar glass cleaners						
fumes from burning wax candles						
odors from dry-garbage incinerators						

ASPHALTS, TARS, RESINS, and DYES

	Love or crave	Dislike or hate	Made sick by	Feel good from	Feel neutral about	Frequent exposure to
fumes from tarred roofs and roads						
asphalt pavements in hot weather						
tar-containing soaps, shampoos, and ointments						
odors of ink, carbon paper, typewriter ribbons, and stencils						
dyes in clothing and shoes						
dyes in cosmetics (lipstick, mascara, rouge, powder, other)						

Disinfectants, Deodorants, and Detergents

	Love or crave	Dislike or hate	Made sick by	Feel good from	Feel neutral about	Frequent exposure to
odor of public or household disinfectants and deodorants						
odor of phenol (carbolic acid) or Lysol						
phenol-containing lotions or ointments						
injectable materials containing phenol as a preservative						
fumes from burning creosote-treated wood (railroad ties)						
household detergents						

Miscellaneous

air conditioning						
ammonia fumes						
odor of mothballs						
odor of insect-repellant candles						
odor of termite-extermination treatment						
odor of DDT-containing insecticide sprays						
odor of chlordane, lindane, parathion, dieldrin, or other insecticide sprays						

	Love or crave	Dislike or hate	Made sick by	Feel good from	Feel neutral about	Frequent exposure to
odor of the fruit and vegetable sections of supermarkets						
odor of chlorinated water						
drinking of chlorinated water						
fumes of chlorine gas						
odor of Chlorox and other hypochlorite bleaches						
fumes from sulfur-processing plants						
fumes of sulfur dioxide						

Pine

	Love or crave	Dislike or hate	Made sick by	Feel good from	Feel neutral about	Frequent exposure to
odor of Christmas trees and other indoor evergreen decorations						
odor of knotty-pine interiors						
odor from sanding or working with pine or cedar wood						
odor of cedar-scented furniture polish						
odor of pine-scented household deodorants						

	Love or crave	Dislike or hate	Made sick by	Feel good from	Feel neutral about	Frequent exposure to
odor of pine-scented bath oils, shampoos, or soaps						
odor of turpentine or turpentine-containing paints						
odor of burning pine cones or wood						

The greater the intensity of your reaction to a given chemical substance, the more likely you are to be susceptible or allergic to it. With very little study of their responses to this questionnaire, chemically susceptible arthritics will realize that their arthritis (and perhaps many other unrecognized ecologic ailments) flares up when they are exposed to many of the commonly encountered, biologically active chemical substances that are part of twentieth century living.

Chemical Questionnaire C

Now we'll examine your environment. Please answer the following questions from my office questionnaire.

Please check if you are exposed to any of the following:

	Your home	Your job	In school	In other places (name them)
gas appliances:				
water heater				
stove				
dryer				
heating system				
dog(s)				
cat(s)				
other animal(s)				
tobacco smoke				
yours				
others				
chemical odors/solvents				
insect sprays/exterminator				
dampness problems				
dust				
potted plants				
mildew/molds/musty odor				
paint/gasoline				
pollution				
agricultural chemicals				

*Home Environment**

Please check for answer.

My home is a single family dwelling___ Owned___ Rented ___
  two-family dwelling___ Owned___ Rented___
  an apartment___ Owned___ Rented___ Shared___
  other_____

Does a family member have a workshop/hobby room in the home?
  Yes___ No___

*This tells you that you may or may not be in control of your environment and whether you can make changes to improve the environment you have great exposure to.

Heating system has an oil furnace?___
　　gas furnace?___
　　electric heat? (floor___ wall___ ceiling___ baseboard___)
　　hot-air heat? (register and ducts)___
　　hot-water heat? (radiator/pipes)___
　　wood-burning stove?___
　　fireplaces?___
　　no heat?___
　　other?___
Where is the furnace of the heating system located:
　　basement___
　　crawl space___
　　on the first floor___
　　next to the kitchen___
　　next to the living room___
　　next to the bathroom___
　　next to a bedroom___
Is there a fuel-oil storage tank in the basement? Yes___ No___
If yes, is the odor of oil noted after oil has been delivered? Yes___
　　No___
If yes, does the odor remain for a few days?___ a week___, longer
　　than a week?___ is always detectable?___
Is some fuel oil spilled in the basement? Yes___ No___, or
　　on the ground next to the house when it is delivered? Yes___
　　No___
Do you have a garage? Yes___ No___
Do garage odors or fumes from the garage enter your home? Yes___
　　No___
Is the garage attached to___ beneath___ or not attached to___ your
　　home/apartment building?
Are you uncomfortable in the garage? Yes___ No___
　　Describe:_____
Please check garage location:
　　under the patient's bedroom___
　　under another bedroom___
　　under other room___
　　opens into kitchen___
　　opens into laundry room___
　　opens into family room___
　　attached by breezeway___
　　underground garage___
　　not used to park car___
　　other:_____

Beneath the house, is there a basement?___
   crawl space?___
   neither?___
Is the basement floor made of dirt?___ concrete?___
Is the crawl-space floor made of dirt?___ concrete?___ both?___
Is the basement wet?___ damp?___ dry?___ always?___ at times?___
Is the crawl space wet?___ damp?___dry?___ always?___ at times?___
Do you use a pump to keep the basement/crawl space dry? Yes___
   No___
Is your home built on a cement slab? Yes___ No___
Does the home have a cellar with a dirt floor? Yes___ No___
What is stored in the cellar, workshop, or garage?

	cellar	workshop	garage
car_____	_____	_____	_____
lawn mower_____	_____	_____	_____
gasoline_____	_____	_____	_____
paint_____	_____	_____	_____
garden and lawn chemicals_____	_____	_____	_____
carpet/rugs_____	_____	_____	_____
newspapers/magazines_____	_____	_____	_____
books_____	_____	_____	_____
clothing_____	_____	_____	_____
other:	_____	_____	_____

Is the area around the home damp and/or swampy all the time?
   Yes_____ No_____
   Only when it rains? Yes_____ No_____
Is the home in open sunshine?_____
   completely shaded?_____
   partly shaded?_____
   surrounded by many trees?_____
   surrounded by other buildings?_____
Do you see any mold or mildew in any part of the house?
   Yes_____ No_____
   Where:
Is there any odor of mold or mildew in the home? Yes_____
   No_____
   Where:
Is dehumidifier necessary in the home all the time?_____
   occasionally?_____
   seasonally?_____
   never used?_____

Which rooms or areas need a dehumidifier?_____

Is the house very dry?_____ very dusty?_____

Is there a dusty odor in the home? Yes_____ No_____
　Where:_____

Are you uncomfortable in any particular room or part of your
　home? Yes_____ No_____ Check the location.
　attic_____ basement/cellar_____ garage_____
　kitchen_____ dining room_____ entrance_____
　your bedroom_____ other bedroom_____ hallway_____
　living room_____ family room_____
　laundry room_____ pantry_____ utility/storage
　　room_____
　workshop/hobby room_____

Chemical Exposures

　Please check the following where appropriate.

Your residence is near _____ is on _____ a heavily traveled road.
　Describe:_____

Are there any factories nearby (within a mile radius of the home)?
　Yes __ No __

How close to the home is the nearest industrial center discharging
　smoke or fumes into the air?

Do any fumes reach your home from local traffic __ or local
　industry __
　No odors noted __

Do you notice these odors outdoors? __ indoors? __

Do these odors cause any symptoms? Yes __ No __
　If yes, describe:_____

Do you notice any odor when you drive past these industrial
　centers/factories? Yes __ No __
　If yes, describe:_____

Does any member of your family have a home occupation that
　brings in or generates chemical odors in the home?
　Yes __ No __
　If yes, describe:_____

Do you or any family member have hobbies that employ odorous
　glues, paints, or chemicals of any kind (model kits, chemistry
　sets, photographic equipment, etc.) Yes __ No __
　If yes, please identify: _____

Does your home have a peculiar or characteristic odor?
Yes __ No __
If yes, describe:_____

Does any family member bring residual chemical fumes __ or
tobacco smoke odor __ into the home on the clothing he or she
wears during working hours? Yes __ No __
If yes, describe:_____

Do you find that many odors are unpleasant to you? Yes __ No __
Do they make you ill or bring on familiar symptoms? Yes __ No __
Do you easily detect odors that other people may not notice? Yes
__ No __
Do you detect various odors before other people may be aware of
them? Yes __ No __
If yes, which odors:
leaking gas __
perfumes __
smoke __
mold __
other:

Does your job expose you to chemical agents, odors, or fumes?
Yes __ No __ Constantly __ Frequently __ Occasionally __
If yes, to which chemicals: _____
Describe your job:

Are you bothered by __ or feel ill __ at work from a job-associated
exposure? Yes __ No __
List the substances _____

Has any previous employment exposed you to chemical agents
and/or odors or fumes? Yes __ No __
If yes, how long were you exposed and to what:

In the past were you ill __ or bothered by __ chemicals, odors or
fumes?
Describe _____

Have any of your co-workers complained of work
environment–related symptoms? Yes __ No __

Do you feel better at home toward the end of your weekend?
Yes __ No __

Do you gradually __ or immediately __
become uncomfortable __ or ill __
after returning to work on Monday?

Summary of Common Chemical Exposures

Please check the response you usually have after an exposure to the following:

	No re-action	Like	Dis-like	Love	Hate	Feel Good	Feel Sick	Frequent Exposure
tobacco smoke								
hair spray								
fresh paint								
paint thinner								
natural gas—leaking								
natural gas—burning (oven, stove, furnace)								
auto exhaust								
truck and bus fumes (diesel)								
furniture polish								
floor wax								
new plastic (shower curtain, tablecloth)								
cologne								
perfume								
aftershave lotion								
air freshener								
disinfectants (Lysol, Pinesol, etc.)								
swimming-pool odor								
household detergent (floor, laundry, dishes)								
permanent magic marker								
deodorant (spray, bar, roll-on)								
Clorox/Ajax/Comet (bleach)								
insect sprays/exterminator								

	No re-action	Like	Dis-like	Love	Hate	Feel Good	Feel Sick	Frequent Exposure
gasoline/kerosene/fuel oil								
freshly printed material (from copier/ ditto machine) (papers/magazines)								
new-car odor								
dry-goods or textile stores								
dry-cleaning store or fluid								
oven cleaner								
cosmetics								
beauty parlor/ barber shop								
florist								
roofing tar								
freshly tarred road								
fresh blacktop								
new rubber								
adhesive/mastic floor coverings								

With all the preceding answers that you have given in mind, I want you to sharpen your diagnostic focus. Please carefully review this chapter, in detail. Note all the items that affect you and be aware of the substances with which you have regular contact at home, in transit, on the job, and elsewhere. Circle in red every substance that causes or has caused arthritis symptoms.

Keep in mind that chemically sensitive people often have a very keen sense of smell and are able to detect even faint odors of substances that many others miss completely or just barely notice. These chemically susceptible individuals are the ones who smell leaking gas when others do not and repeatedly phone the gas company to repair leaks that the service man cannot find for weeks or months before another more sensitive employee finds it. They can tell if a room was painted a week ago or if someone wearing perfume was in the room several hours ago. Many dust- and mold-allergic persons also detect the presence of airborne allergens before non-allergics do.

Your allergies to inhalant particles and your chemical sensitivities should be fairly obvious to you by now. A *yes* item in Section A or a highly reactive substance in Section B which is also circled for an arthritis response or checked for frequent contact may be an important factor in the causation of your arthritis symptoms.

Check Yourself

You can test your arthritis response to chemicals with the same general techniques you used for food testing. First you will "fast" in a chemical sense through an environmental cleanup, and then you will test.

You go on a chemical fast by eliminating as many possible and probable chemical offenders from your environment as thoroughly as possible. The first substances to remove are those highly probable ones you pinpointed in your questionnaires. They are the ones most likely to evoke an arthritic reaction when you are ready to begin your chemical testing. You may not be able completely to eliminate all of them, but there are ways to reduce your exposure to them greatly, at least for the short time required by the test. For instance, if you are very susceptible to petroleum substances and you cannot take time off from work or from your usual errands, find alternate routes that are not heavily trafficked in order to avoid exposure to exhaust fumes as much as possible.

Or if the molds or mildew in your home affect you, spend a mold-free week in a friend's home or a motel that is dry and clean and passes your inspection for visible molds and mold odors. Eat no foods that contain mold products, yeast, or yeast products and fermented substances: bakery goods, cheese, alcoholic beverages, mushrooms, vinegars, and tofu.

If pine groves, pollens, or other natural substances apparently affect you and you live surrounded by them in the country, remain inside an air-conditioned residence with air that has passed through particle-catching filters or arrange to spend time in another home or in an apartment or a hotel in the city or on the beach.

No matter what your suspected sensitivities, conduct your environmental chemical cleanup thoroughly in these basic ways:

Do as complete a job as possible. Do *not* use commercial cleaning products! Instead, vacuum everything—floors, rugs, baseboards, upholstered furniture, bric-a-brac, draperies, even walls. When you are done, discard the bag (or bags!) full of dust. If possible, send curtains, draperies, and rugs to the cleaner, to be picked up and thoroughly aired after your testing period, or wash them in natural soaps like Ivory, Rokeach, or Arm & Hammer washing soda.

Remove as many chemical products as possible from your home. Get rid of spray cans and any open containers of anything chemical in nature—cleaning agents, paints, cosmetics, aerosol cans, all toiletries and medications (except for those you must take by prescription on a continuing basis). Store all these elsewhere or seal them in an out-of-the-way cupboard or in large plastic bags in the garage or basement. Turn off all gas and oil and use electricity for cooking and heating temporarily. Park the car outside a connected garage.

Clear out *any* substance that has a distinctive odor. Make a room-to-room "sniff search" of your home and put away anything that you can smell, whether you like or dislike the odor, whether or not anyone else in the household can smell it. Seal off with tape and/or weather stripping a damp-smelling basement or a musty-smelling attic after doing your best to make it dry and clean. Get help if these areas of your home make you uncomfortable in any way.

If possible, use only natural fibers during your testing period: cotton towels and sheets and folded cotton towels or blankets inside a cotton pillowcase for a pillow; cotton or (unless you know wool causes problems) woolen clothing. Natural materials like silk and linen are usually tolerated. Polyesters and other synthetics are petroleum based and should be avoided. Select the oldest natural-fiber clothing and linens from your closet and wash them in Ivory, Rokeach, or Arm & Hammer. Seal the rest in a separate closet for the duration of your "fast." Remove any plastic covers from your mattress or any other furniture. If your mattress is made of plastic or artificial foam, cover it with clean blankets beneath your cotton sheets. Plastic and foam rubber are also petroleum based (as, by the way, are the insulators around the wires in electric blankets), so you will want to do without them temporarily.

Because plastic can pose a problem, also put away any

plastic or Teflon-lined kitchen utensils. Instead, cook with Pyrex, cast iron, stainless steel, enamel, or Corningware. Store foods and beverages in glass containers. Don't cook in aluminum pans; many people are sensitive to foods cooked in aluminum. Clean dishes in natural soaps; use baking soda for all scouring.

As for food itself, see the diet chapters for advice. Although you need not be on a strict fast during your chemical-test period, you should eat only those foods that you know are compatible with your system and obtain foods that you know are as pure (free of chemical additives and contaminants) as possible. Preservatives, synthetic flavors and artificial coloring, and food-processing agents are chemicals to be avoided. In order to minimize the residual chemicals that are already present in your body from many years of previous exposure to various biologically active chemical substances, you should eat pure, fresh foods and drink only bottled-in-glass spring water, which does not contain the chemicals of tap water from a municipal water-treatment plant or the body of water from which your supply is obtained. Of course, for the duration of the test—and hopefully thereafter—you will not smoke and will not allow tobacco smoke in your home. The use of all types of odorous household chemicals is to be avoided.

Tobacco smoke is a complex mixture of chemical fumes that is generated by the combustion of many substances—some toxic—that come from several sources. They include the nicotine- and cadmium-containing tobacco plant itself; the persistent residues of agrochemicals used in tobacco-crop production (insecticides, fungicides, herbicides, fertilizer); the various agents used for curing, flavoring, and imparting specific aromas to the tobacco leaf; and the chemically treated paper that cigarettes are rolled in.

If your arthritis is caused by or aggravated by an internal state of chemical susceptibility to tobacco smoke that involves your joints and their surrounding structures, smoking may be a major factor in your arthritis. The fumes that you inhale will pass through the thin walls of the microscopic air sacs in your lungs (the alveoli), enter the bloodstream, and be transported throughout your body to every vulnerable structure. Upon contact with some components of smoke, these vulnerable areas may become the sites of adverse arthritis reactions.

The negative effects of smoking may require several weeks to clear from your system, and this is why the full benefit of discontinuing this harmful activity will not be apparent immediately, although you will probably begin to feel better as soon as your continuous exposure to the combustion fumes is stopped.

To cleanse the "outside" of you: use only simple, "natural," unscented or lightly scented soaps like Ivory or Rokeach,* Castile, Neutrogena, or Johnson's Baby Shampoo in conjunction with spring water (not tap water!), which you can heat for sponge baths. Shave with an electric razor or use a regular razor with unscented soap; if an astringent is necessary, use iced spring water. Brush your teeth with sea salt or baking soda along with spring water. If you are concerned about personal odor, baking soda makes an excellent and safe deodorant dusting powder or mouthwash. Wear no makeup, perfume, aftershave lotion, or other scented "chemical" cosmetics during the test period. If you feel the need, explain to your friends what you are doing, so that they will understand why you don't look and smell the way you usually do in your "regular" chemical package (don't worry—they'll love you anyway!).

Finally, love them though you do, board your pets and plants elsewhere during this testing period. Pet danders, saliva, and odors are among the most common allergic offenders. Don't worry if your pet is a prime suspect behind your arthritis— measures other than giving it away are available to you. And the soil of your potted plants can be a reservoir of huge numbers of many species of allergically potent molds that may be a factor in your arthritis.

Follow this life-style for ten days.

This preparation is not as complicated as it may seem at first reading. And even if you think it sounds like too much trouble, think again about the pain you have been suffering from your arthritis and the many things that you are unable to do and would love to do. If it is necessary for you to take a little trouble—or make a major effort— to find out what is presently causing that pain and might lead to possible crippling in the future, whom are you doing this for? Let's find and then eliminate the identifiable causes of your arthritis and get you as well as you can be. Of course it's worth it. Be your own

---

*Ivory soap is lightly perfumed and there are some chemically sensitive people who cannot tolerate it.

best friend. Extra effort at home may make it possible for some individuals to do the job at home instead of having to travel to an ecology unit a considerable distance away.

Even with all this preparation and chemical fasting at home, you will encounter potential arthritis triggers outside your home. But by reducing as much as possible the levels of indoor chemical pollutants that affect you most, you will do a lot toward immediately feeling better as well as preparing your system to react to the direct tests that follow—just as you did when you were fasting or eliminating offenders prior to testing foods. Remember, while it is possible to test for both foods and chemicals at the same time, as we do under near-laboratory conditions in the hospital-based environmentally controlled ecologic units at bioecologic centers, you will find it easier to check them out separately when you are doing it on your own. The chemical cleanup done before food testing, along with the inhalant cleanup, will give better results with the food tests, and with the chemicals and inhalants gone, you will undoubtedly feel better.

After you have been on your chemical fast for at least one week— and ten days is better (chemicals already in you take longer to clear than food because they are locked in "tighter" and leave your system slowly)—begin to reintroduce chemicals into your system. The test schedule (pp. 212–214) will give you an idea of how to go about it, but you should choose some of your own prime suspects to test by selecting from the items you rated highest in the questionnaire section of this chapter.

If you know that certain odors, fumes, and vapors of chemical origin really do bother you in many ways, you can take one of the few commonsense shortcuts that I do not object to at all. Clean up that house chemically from cellar to attic and don't forget the garage. Do as good a job as is humanly possible. Get everything!

You may be so susceptible to chemicals—so highly allergic to your chemical environment of petroleum-derived solvents and synthetic indoor air pollutants—that it is not medically wise for you to do this essential job yourself. One of the best financial investments you can make for that body you live in is to hire someone who is not chemically susceptible to do a carefully supervised A-1 job that may perform a miracle for you.

It may also do something very special for other members of your family—something great! No one ever knew that X, Y, or Z, your relatives living in the same unhealthy, technologically polluted environment that you call home, were also chemical victims. Your personal search for better health may bring about a spectacular unanticipated bonus—X, Y, and Z, all of them, may soon start to feel much better in different ways: more energy and smiling; dizzy spells and headaches gone; more alert; better concentration and memory that may cause a learning disability to vanish; assorted aches and pains diminished or gone . . . I think you have the idea by now.

When your review of past and present observations of your responses to the complex chemical environment of modern living has positively identified you as a chemically susceptible individual, you must go all out to make your home an ecologically sound haven. It is very desirable that you create an oasis in which you will be as free as possible from the factors in your environment that have been making you ill and really are not good for anyone's health even if no one else presently seems to be affected by these substances. Even a one-room oasis in a "safe" home can be very effective.

You have my word that the home-wide commonsense shortcut to making a safer, better chemical environment often works very well without your having to do a single chemical test. If you are very curious and must see for yourself, do the self-testing for chemical susceptibility very gently—go easy on yourself. Expose yourself to small amounts of test materials for the shortest interval of time as is required to show clearly that the substances being investigated are bad for you. Don't be a stubborn or foolish junior scientist. *Stop testing as soon as you have learned enough.* It is not using common sense to do otherwise. Why get sick or make yourself more uncomfortable than necessary to establish the role of any chemical offender?

What have you learned? If, according to the recorded responses on your chart, any of the chemical odors/fumes tests has produced an arthritis flare-up or any other symptoms, you have learned that allergylike susceptibility to volatile chemicals plays a causative role in your arthritic suffering and/or affects your general health. "Fine! But what can I do about it?" you may ask. Say you react to the fumes of different petroleum products, yet you must live in an automobile-exhaust-filled and otherwise polluted city or drive a car or hold a job at a paint or plastics plant. It may not be absolutely necessary, even though it may be highly advisable, for you to move or quit your job. If you use your ingenuity in the ways suggested on pages 207–209 to reduce the level of petroleum-derived products in your home, you may be able to increase your tolerance to them (raise your threshold) to a point at which you can cope to a limited degree

Tests for Chemical Susceptibility (within the limits of your tolerance)

Test one chemical when you first get up in the morning, another in midafternoon, and a third in the early evening, if it is not too much of a stress for you to do so.

Day #1

Chlorine in Drinking Water

Drink 3 glasses of chlorine-treated tap water from your kitchen or bathroom sink (your usual source).

Furniture Polish

Spray your furniture polish on a rag until it is soaked. Sit two feet away in a small room for 15–20 minutes with the door shut unless symptoms appear before 15 minutes elapse.

Ammonia

Mix 1 tablespoon in 1 cup of spring water. Soak a 3×3-inch piece of blotter and place it on a plate. Then sit two feet away in a small room for up to 20 minutes if that much time is required to show that symptoms will not develop. As soon as important symptoms begin to make their appearance, discontinue your ammonia exposure and record your observations.

Day #2

Clorox/Chlorine Bleach

Mix 1 tablespoon in 1 cup of water. Soak a blotter and sit two feet away in a small room for up to 15–20 minutes with the door shut. Follow the ammonia instructions from Day #1.

Cigar

Light three cigars (do not smoke them) and put them in an ashtray. Sit two feet away in a small room for 15–20 minutes or less with the door shut.

Moth Flakes

Put 1 teaspoon in an empty can. Sit two feet away in a small room for 15–20 minutes if necessary.

Day #3
Detergent

Fill the bathroom sink with a laundry detergent and spring water. Make suds. Stay in the bathroom for 15–20 minutes.

Day #4
Cigarettes

Light three cigarettes (do not smoke them) and put them in an ashtray. Sit two feet away in a small room for 15–20 minutes with the door shut.

Day #5
Combustion Fumes from a Lighted Gas Stove

Turn on the oven and all the burners; keep the oven door open. Close or seal off the kitchen door, close the windows, and sit in the kitchen for 15–20 minutes or less if you have symptoms before 15 minutes have elapsed.

Fresh Newsprint

Buy a freshly printed newspaper and read it for 15–20 minutes or less. Hold it close to you.

Hair Spray

Spray hair spray for 15 seconds in a small room. Stay there for 15–20 minutes or less with the door shut.

Turpentine

Soak a blotter and sit two feet away in a small room for 15–20 minutes or less with the door shut.

Diesel or Gasoline Exhaust Fumes

Sit on a chair in your driveway five to ten feet behind your car with the motor running (brakes locked and gearshift in park position). Remain in the chair for up to 20 minutes.

Foam Rubber

Lie down for 15–20 minutes or less with your head on a new foam-rubber pillow or plastic foam pillow (use the kind you usually sleep on).

Perfume/Cologne

Take your favorite perfume or cologne and place a few drops on a piece of cloth or blotter paper just under your nose for 15–20 minutes or less.

Record your chemical reactions on this chart.

	Item tested & reaction	Item tested & reaction	Item tested & reaction
Day 1			
Day 2			
Day 3			
Day 4			
Day 5			

with the other arthritis-inducing factors in your life. Be warned in advance that you may be helped considerably but develop only a limited tolerance.

Or if pollens are a problem and you live in the suburbs or in the country, you might invest in an air-filtration and -conditioning system to protect your home environment from those native airborne allergens during the seasons when they are prevalent. Mold-allergic people may have to remove all the potted plants from their homes; molds grow very well at room temperature in moist soil.

Mold or mildew sensitive? Clean out, air out, and scrub that basement and install a dehumidifier! You may have to heat a cool basement that becomes damp in the summer. Remove mold-covered items.

Pet lovers may be allergic to their pets and yet not be able to give them up. In that case, desensitizing treatments such as those described in Chapter 11 are available, and it is possible that by reducing the overall level of arthritis-inducing substances in your life, you may find that you are able to live comfortably with the dander, saliva, and odors produced by Tabby or Fido.

Likewise, you may have learned that you are sensitive to chemical agents associated with your job. That does not always mean that you must immediately change careers, because if you eliminate as many chemical substances from your daily life as you possibly can, you may raise your overall threshold to the point where you can better tolerate the still undesirable and best avoided on-the-job chemical incitants. Of course, you can also exert "political" pressure to move, remove, or control substances—from tobacco smoke to fumes from open cans or vats of materials—that are hazardous to yourself and others in your work place. It is a fact of life that most individuals with a severe degree of chemical sensitivity need to change jobs associated with moderate to heavy chemical exposures to relieve allergic arthritis and other manifestations of chemical allergy.

Before you take such a drastic step, no matter what you have found your allergies to be, I would strongly recommend that you protect your interests by a visit to a well-trained and experienced clinical ecologist (or bioecologic specialist) for a comprehensive professional evaluation of your problem and counseling regarding your future employment and activities.

In the same vein, some arthritis sufferers may feel that the only way to escape the mildew, pollens, exhaust fumes, or other pollutants that trigger their allergy is to move out of their homes or communities. But you have many alternatives to that big step: by eliminating all potential allergens from your home, you can create an ecologically safe oasis to rest in, where you can recuperate and hopefully build up your resistance. Even people with no specific chemical sensitivities will benefit from such an environment because of all the types of damage that the chemicals in our surroundings can create throughout one's body. Repairing and remodeling your present home are often less costly solutions than selling a home and buying a new one, since there will be two substantial real estate commissions as well as moving expenses and the inevitable and not inconsiderable costs of some redecorating and repairs, and possibly a few pieces of new furniture will be needed.

10

The Lifetime Arthritis-Relief Diet

This chapter will show you how it may be possible to keep many of the substances that cause your arthritis at levels considerably lower than your threshold for developing symptoms. If you are successful, you will be able to tolerate some—and perhaps a large number—of the presently uncontrolled foods, airborne allergens, and chemical incitants that are causing your arthritis and may also have other negative effects on your physical and mental health.

First, you need to determine your overall sensitivities and your tolerance for dietary factors—the current state of your food allergies. You will do this systematically by gradually adding to the group of foods that you have already tested by means of your just-completed series of single-food challenges in your rotary diet. During what I call Phase One of the Lifetime Arthritis Relief Diet, you will continue to eat one "new" (untested) food per meal until you have observed the effects of the entire range of foods that is currently available to you. One at a time, additional foods will be incorporated in the rotating schedule of foods that you already know you can tolerate.

While you are doing this, you must do everything that is necessary to keep your environment free of those substances to which, as you learned in the last chapter, you are sensitive—and those common offenders that should be controlled or avoided as a preventive measure even if they presently appear to be tolerated.

The Lifetime Arthritis-Relief Diet: Phase One

Review all your rotary diet single-food test results to date. Then study the comprehensive classification of plant and animal foods beginning on page 157, and the special lists of plant and animal foods on pages 164–165 in which every food belongs to a different biologic family. Select a group of twenty-one additional foods to be studied in a new seven-day rotary diversified diet. Have a high-protein (animal-source) food each evening and work out a suitable morning cereal-and-fruit plan for breakfast and a vegetable and/or fruit plan for your lunches. If you wish, there is no reason you cannot have a high-protein food for breakfast or lunch.

Repeat this new group of twenty-one foods at least one time (an additional 7-day cycle) to confirm your sensitivities as well as your tolerance to the nonreaction-causing foods in this group, and, once again, observe the effects of those foods that caused only mild symptoms and may be included in your diet.

Now you have added more foods to your "safe" list and your offenders list, and you can repeat this procedure with another group of twenty-one foods. This will increase the number of available safe foods as well as give you another opportunity to discover additional foods that affect your arthritis (or other conditions).

If your selection of foods is severely limited because your food problem is very bad, you have to work a little harder, but there are other foods. Some foods with almost the same name belong to different families and can be eaten on successive days or even in successive meals. The relationship between such foods must be carefully checked before you include them in your diet. For example, California halibut is in a different family from Atlantic halibut. Summer flounder and southern flounder belong to the same family, but winter flounder and right-eyed flounder belong to another family. Yellow perch and white perch belong to different families. There are two different bass families, and there are many shark families. Study the classification very carefully; check the ethnic food stores, and do not overlook the game meats.

When you have carefully investigated the effects of all or most of the foods you would presently like to eat, it is time to try a series of combinations of two foods at each meal. Each combination must be evaluated, because the total effect of two safe foods cannot be predicted even though the individual foods were tolerated when eaten separately. See the sample diet on page 223.

It is not very likely that you will be able to tolerate all the cereal grains, and it is usually not possible to tolerate cereals more often than every forty-eight hours even though they are classified in different tribes of the grass family. Cereals in the same tribe—barley, rye, and wheat—must be rotated on at least a four-day schedule with respect to each other because they are considered to be almost identical in the allergic sense. Members of the same botanic tribe share more features in common than are shared by foods that belong to the same family. Although you might tolerate corn, oats, and rice on Monday, Wednesday, and Friday, respectively—and this is rather close spacing for cereal grains—you should not eat the barley-rye-wheat tribal group on such a schedule.

They require a full four-day spacing, such as Monday-Friday-Tuesday-Saturday, schedule, in order for you to maintain your tolerance to these very closely related foods; they require their own schedule of rotation. You might find it easier to have a single day in your rotation on which you will eat one of these three grains, with barley on Day 1 of Cycle I, rye on Day 1 of Cycle II, and wheat on Day 1 of Cycle III.

The same situation exists for other members of the plant kingdom, including the gourd and the mustard families. Within both of these botanic families are foods that also must be considered to be allergically identical, and identical foods may require a four-day spacing in the rotary diet with respect to each other, whereas the really different ("nonidentical") members within a family can be eaten on alternate days in most instances. In the gourd family, the very closely related (almost allergically identical) members are canteloupe, casaba melon, crenshaw melon, honeydew melon, muskmelon, Persian and Spanish melons. The nonidentical members of this family are cucumber, winter squash,* summer squash† and watermelon. It is very likely that for many allergic persons, the first group of melons must be on a four-day or greater rotation with respect to each of the other melons; the nonidentical gourds will probably be well tolerated on an every-other-day basis.

The same situation, with respect to allergic identity, also applies to the "taste-alike" foods in the mustard family. They are broccoli,

---

*Hubbard, butternut, and acorn squash, and large pumpkin are very similar and should be treated, until proven otherwise, as being allergically identical.

†Summer squash and regular pumpkin, including pumpkin seeds and pumpkin meals, should also be considered as interchangeable, almost identical foods.

brussels sprouts, cabbage (green and red), cauliflower, celery cabbage, collards, kale, and kohlrabi. The other mustard foods—Chinese cabbage, horseradish, mustard (greens and seeds), radish, rutabaga, turnip, and watercress—are sufficiently different from each other (the nonidentical members of this family) to be rotated on a forty-eight-hour schedule.

Recapitulation of Instructions

Do not eat the same food more than once during any five, six, or seven-day period in a rotation cycle. Do not eat foods from the same family more than once every other day. And pay special attention to the foods within a family that are to be treated as allergically identical. By this time you will be very much aware of the foods to which you are allergically sensitive and those foods that do not affect you. Please check the food-family biologic classification charts once more to be sure that you are not making any errors in your selection and schedule.

A sample menu appears on page 224, but you will do best and learn more about food and you by constructing and adding to (and removing from) your own individualized, person-specific test menus. Your selection of the foods to be included in the test menus should be chosen from those foods that seem to be the most likely offenders, foods that appear to be the least hazardous for you, and those you want to try for any reason. And don't worry: no matter how you go about your selection, you will obtain all the information you seek in good time if you are careful—just keep very good records and watch those food families.

Continue this self-selected series of food cycles until you have included foods from all the food families in your diet. Pretty soon you will be able to expand your dietary horizons, and you will be able to experiment with selection and spacing in the future. But for now please be cautious about what you add to your menu and when you eat it. Keep foods and food families separate enough so that you can positively identify which ones are the offenders in case of an allergic arthritis flare-up or the appearance of any other familiar symptoms.

Very soon you will be able to add a variety of seasonings, but you must be sure to include them in or on foods that you have already tested and know you do not react to. See pages 225–230 for kitchen-tested combinations of various foods and the seasonings that go well with them. And pay attention to the botanic family classification and spacing of the herbs, spices, and flavors that you use.

Maintain your records carefully, with strict attention to detail. If you experience a flare-up and you do not know exactly what or when you ate last, as well as where you were and what you did there, you may not have any idea of what caused your difficulties. Without adequate records, there is a very good chance that you, like many others, will forget some important information that you were absolutely certain you would never forget.

However, even in such a situation all is not lost. Much has been gained despite your overloaded and less-than-perfect memory. You will have experienced clinically significant allergic reactions to a number of foods, which have convinced you of the importance of food allergy in your life. Your only problem originating from this situation is, "Which food did what to me?"

By now you have had enough experience with food lists and recordkeeping. This will not be a problem for you but simply a matter of habit. Until you are very much better, you should continue to record your diet and reactions carefully on forms like those on page 183, so that you will always be able to refer to this vital information about those foods that cause reactions and those foods that do not.

The Lifetime Diet: Permanent Phase

You have completed the initial phase and added to your diagnostic menu all those foods to which you know you are not arthritis- or any-other-illness prone, and you have managed the proper separation of foods within the same food families. You are ready to begin the lifetime diet. I'm sure that by now you are not surprised to learn that the lifetime diet does *not* mean that you immediately begin to eat all those foods that were once your favorites.

First, you will gradually incorporate other "safe" foods into your menu. Then, you will go to meals consisting of two-food, three-food, and four-food combinations in a diet that you will prove step by step is well tolerated. And after you have avoided clearly demonstrated offenders and potentially dangerous foods for an adequate biologic rest period, you may begin to add suspect foods to your diet. Then you can perform single-food testing of those foods that once were definite offenders and may now be safe for you if you have avoided them long enough to regain your tolerance to them. The odds are in

Sample 6-Day Rotary Diversified Diet
(Showing one-food meals)

	Day 1	Day 2	Day 3	Day 4	Day 5	Day 6
Breakfast	Pineapple	Corn[1]	Melon[4]	(Oat or Rice)[1]	Grapefruit[5]	Wheat[1]
Lunch	Squash[4]	Sweet Potato	Almond[8]	Mango[17]	Cottage Cheese[10]	Papaya
Dinner	(Lamb or Beef)[10]	(Cod or Haddock)	Chicken[2] or Crab	Flounder or Sole	Pork or Turkey	Tuna or Shrimp

NOTE: Parentheses enclose foods in the same family.

This one-food-a-meal diet is the basis of the two-food-a-meal and three- or four-food-a-meal diets that follow. Foods having the same number belong to the family (note spacing). Select additional foods because of family relationships, and space them to prevent family overloading of foods that are closely related to each other. For instance, almond from family 8 is used for lunch on Day 3 in the one-food-a-meal diet and apricot or peach from family 8 is added to Breakfast on Day 1 in the three- or four-food-a-meal diet. Chicken from family 2 is used at dinner on Day 3 in the one-food-a-meal diet, and egg, also from family 2, is added to breakfast on Day 1 in the two-food-a-meal diet.

Sample 6-Day Rotary Diversified Diet
(Showing two-food meals)

	Day 1	Day 2	Day 3	Day 4	Day 5	Day 6
Breakfast	Pineapple and Egg[2]	Corn[1] and Apple[3]	Melon[4] and Orange[5]	(Oat or Rice)[1] and Banana	Grapefruit[5] and Pear[3]	Wheat[1] and (Prune, Plum or Cherry)[8]
Lunch	Squash[4] and (String Bean or Kidney Bean)[6]	Sweet Potato and (Celery or Parsnip)[7]	Almond[8] and (Peas or Lima Bean)[6]	Mango[17] and (Cauliflower or Cabbage or Broccoli)[9]	Cottage Cheese[10] and Walnuts[12] or (Lentil or Peanut)[6]	Papaya and Rutabaga[9]
Dinner	(Lamb or Beef)[10] and Artichoke[14]	(Cod or Haddock) and Turnip[9]	Chicken[2] or Crab and Lettuce[14]	Flounder or Sole and Potato[13] or Yucca[18]	Pork or Turkey and Carrots[7]	Tuna or Shrimp and Tomato[13]

NOTE: Parentheses enclose foods in the same family. Foods having the same number belong to the same family (note spacing intervals between members of the same family). A second food in each meal has been added to the one-food-a-meal diet. The foods are compatible in terms of family relationships and spacing. This doesn't guarantee that any of these combinations will be tolerated, however, because each new combination must be tested. The following three- or four-food-a-meal diet shows that it is possible to eat well once the rotary diet is established.

Sample Multiple Purpose 6-Day Rotary Diversified Diet
(Showing three-food and four-food meals)

	Day 1	Day 2	Day 3	Day 4	Day 5	Day 6
Breakfast	Pineapple and Egg[2] and (Apricot or Peach)[8]	Corn[1] and Apple[3] and Blueberry or Persimmon	Melon[4] and Orange[5] and Rhubarb[16]	(Oat or Rice)[1] and Banana and (Strawberry or Raspberry)	Grapefruit[5] and Pear[3] and Buckwheat[16]	Wheat[1] and (Prune, Plum or Cherry)[8] and Yam, American
Lunch	Squash[4] and (String Bean or Kidney Bean)[6]	Sweet Potato and (Celery or Parsnip)[7]	Almond[8] and (Peas or Lima Bean)[6]	Mango[17] and (Cauliflower or Cabbage or Broccoli)[9]	Cottage Cheese[10] and Walnuts[12] or (Lentil or Peanut)[6]	Papaya and Rutabaga[9]
Dinner	(Lamb or Beef)[10] and Artichoke[14] and Beets[11] and/or Coconut[15]	(Cod or Haddock) and Turnip[9] and (Eggplant or Pepper)[13] and/or Figs	(Chicken[2] or Crab) and Lettuce[14] and Pecans[12] and/or Dates[15]	(Flounder or Sole) and Potato[13] or Yucca[18] and Brazil Nut and/or Chestnut	Pork or Turkey and Carrots[7] and Sunflower Seed[14] and/or (Watermelon or Cucumber)[4]	Tuna or Shrimp and Tomato[13] and Onion[18] and/or Cashew[17]

NOTE: Parentheses enclose foods in the same family.
Foods having the same number belong to the same family (note spacing intervals between members of the same family).
In some cycles of rotation in the near future, try: milk, grape, haddock, lobster, scallops, soy, chocolate, sugar, onion, garlic, black pepper, etc.

Herbs and Spices for Meats, Poultry, and Seafood

The herb and spice charts are designed to show you at a glance many food-herb-spice combinations. Foods are listed across the top of the chart and herbs and spices are listed in the column on the left. Taste-test research has been done to determine which herbs and spices taste best with each food. You will find a delicious combination of food and herb or spice where there is an X in the box where the herb or spice and food join. Be sure to rotate the herbs and spices properly as you use them with your rotation of foods.

Reprinted from *Dr. Mandell's Allergy-Free Cook Book*, by Fran Gare Mandell, with the permission of Simon and Schuster, publishers of Pocket Books.

Herbs	Beef	Pork	Lamb	Veal	Game Meats	Chicken and Turkey	Game Birds	Eggs	Fish	Shellfish
Allspice	X	X			X					
Anise	X		X							X
Basil	X	X		X				X	X	X
Bay Leaf	X	X	X	X	X	X	X		X	X
Caraway	X	X	X	X	X	X	X		X	
Cardamom		X	X		X	X	X			
Cayenne	X	X	X	X	X	X	X	X	X	X
Celery seed	X	X	X	X	X	X	X	X	X	X
Chili powder	X				X			X		
Chives				X		X		X	X	X
Cinnamon	X	X			X					
Clove	X									
Coriander	X	X		X	X	X	X			
Cumin	X	X	X	X	X	X	X	X	X	X
Dill	X					X	X	X	X	X
Garlic	X	X	X	X	X	X	X	X	X	X
Ginger	X	X	X	X	X	X	X			

Herbs	Beef	Pork	Lamb	Veal	Game Meats	Chicken and Turkey	Game Birds	Eggs	Fish	Shellfish
Horseradish	X	X	X	X	X	X	X			
Leeks	X	X	X	X	X	X	X	X	X	X
Mace		X			X		X			
Marjoram		X	X	X						
Mint			X							
Mustard	X	X	X	X	X	X	X	X	X	X
Nutmeg	X			X		X	X			
Onion	X	X	X							
Oregano	X	X	X	X	X	X	X		X	X
Paprika	X	X	X	X	X	X	X	X	X	X
Parsley	X	X	X							
Pepper	X	X	X	X	X	X	X	X	X	X
Poppy						X			X	
Rosemary	X	X	X	X	X	X	X	X	X	X
Sage		X		X	X	X	X			
Savory										
Scallions	X	X	X	X	X	X	X	X	X	X
Sesame	X	X	X	X	X	X	X			
Shallots	X	X	X	X	X	X	X	X	X	X
Tarragon			X			X	X	X	X	X
Thyme	X	X	X	X	X	X	X		X	X
Turmeric		X	X		X	X	X		X	X

Herbs and Spices for Vegetables

Herbs	Artichokes	Asparagus	Beans	Beets	Broccoli	Cabbage	Cauliflower	Carrots	Celery	Corn
Allspice			X		X	X			X	
Anise						X	X	X	X	X
Basil			X		X			X	X	
Bay Leaf	X		X		X		X	X	X	
Caraway				X		X		X	X	
Cardamom			X					X		X
Cayenne	X	X	X		X	X	X	X	X	X
Celery seed	X	X	X	X	X	X	X	X	X	X
Chili powder			X			X			X	X
Chives	X	X	X	X	X	X	X	X	X	X
Cinnamon						X		X		
Clove			X	X		X		X		X
Coriander	X						X	X	X	X
Cumin		X			X		X	X	X	X
Dill	X	X	X	X	X			X	X	X
Garlic	X	X	X	X	X	X	X		X	X
Ginger		X	X	X	X	X	X	X	X	X
Horseradish		X	X	X	X	X				
Leeks		X			X			X		
Mace								X		X

Herbs	Artichokes	Asparagus	Beans	Beets	Broccoli	Cabbage	Cauliflower	Carrots	Celery	Corn
Marjoram			X					X	X	
Mint			X					X		
Mustard		X			X	X	X	X	X	
Nutmeg		X			X			X		
Onion	X	X	X	X	X	X	X	X	X	X
Oregano	X	X	X						X	
Paprika		X		X	X	X	X	X	X	X
Parsley	X	X	X	X	X	X	X	X	X	X
Pepper	X	X	X	X	X	X	X	X	X	X
Poppy		X					X	X	X	
Rosemary			X					X	X	
Sage			X					X		X
Savory			X			X		X		
Scallions	X	X	X	X	X	X	X	X	X	X
Sesame		X	X	X	X	X	X	X	X	
Shallots	X	X	X	X	X	X	X	X	X	X
Tarragon					X			X		
Thyme		X				X	X	X	X	
Turmeric						X	X	X		

Herbs	Cucumber	Eggplant	Mushrooms	Peas	Peppers	Potatoes	Spinach	Squash	Tomatoes
Allspice	X	X					X		X
Anise									X
Basil	X	X	X	X	X	X		X	X
Bay Leaf		X	X		X				X
Caraway	X					X		X	
Cardamom		X	X	X	X	X	X	X	X
Cayenne	X	X	X		X	X	X		X
Celery seed	X	X	X	X	X	X	X	X	X
Chili powder	X	X	X		X	X			X
Chives	X	X	X	X	X	X	X	X	X
Cinnamon									X
Clove	X	X							
Coriander	X	X	X		X	X	X	X	
Cumin	X	X	X	X	X	X			X
Dill	X	X	X	X	X	X		X	X
Garlic	X	X	X	X	X	X	X		X
Ginger	X	X	X	X	X	X	X	X	
Horseradish						X			X
Leeks									
Mace	X					X			

Herbs	Cucumber	Eggplant	Mushrooms	Peas	Peppers	Potatoes	Spinach	Squash	Tomatoes
Marjoram	X				X	X			X
Mint	X			X					X
Mustard	X	X	X		X	X	X		X
Nutmeg							X		
Onion	X	X	X	X	X	X	X	X	X
Oregano		X	X		X	X		X	X
Paprika	X	X	X	X	X	X	X	X	
Parsley	X	X	X	X	X	X	X	X	X
Pepper	X	X	X	X	X	X	X	X	X
Poppy								X	
Rosemary			X	X		X			X
Sage									X
Savory			X					X	X
Scallions	X	X	X	X	X	X	X	X	X
Sesame	X	X	X		X	X	X	X	X
Shallots	X	X	X	X	X	X	X	X	X
Tarragon	X	X	X		X	X	X		X
Thyme		X				X			X
Turmeric				X					X

your favor, and most of my readers will be able to eat at least fifty percent of the foods that used to make them ill.

Once you have thoroughly cleared your system of an offending food by avoiding it and given your body a six- to twelve-week (or longer) rest period, you may tolerate that substance in moderate quantities that are well spaced in your diet without causing arthritis or other symptoms. But you must not do it willy-nilly. Gradually add single foods to each meal of your rotation menu plan, keeping the members within food families properly separated from each other by at least forty-eight hours or longer, as previously instructed.

Do not eat the same food more than once in a rotation of five to seven days or longer. A six-day diet makes every-other-day (48-hour) rotation within biologic families very easy, and an eight-day diet gives a longer rest period before a food is repeated. Some food-allergic individuals do better with longer cycles. I have had a few patients who definitely felt better on nine-, ten-, and twelve-day cycles. A seven-day diet is very convenient because foods are always eaten on the same day of the week, and this is easy to remember.

It has been my clinical experience that within three weeks to three to six months after being completely free of potent food allergens, a patient can tolerate many of the foods that would have caused a severe allergic flare-up in the past. Therefore, three times a week or every other day you may try a different allergic food offender taking small portions at first. Try a group of your all-time-favorite foods. If any food precipitates an arthritis response—even a mild one—or other symptoms, avoid it for a few more weeks and try it again. If it still causes trouble, wait a few months and retest. If it still causes symptoms after two or three months, eliminate that food for a full six months, and if it causes arthritis symptoms again, you know that you have a fixed or permanent intolerance to that food and should avoid it. I know that following rotary diets and food avoidance can be a little difficult for some, but think about the years of chronic pain your arthritis has caused you, and the definite possibility of crippling in the future, and it's very easy to decide which sacrifice is better. You cannot treat your fixed food allergies without professional assistance. But there are several types of medical and allergy treatments by which some of these allergies can be successfully managed if you need or would like to add some more foods to your diet.

When you are thoroughly familiar with the system, you will not need to keep records in order to follow your Lifetime Arthritis Relief program, but you will need to remember some basic principles.

The goal is to keep food allergens from building up to symptom-evoking levels in the body. This is accomplished by ingesting only tolerated quantities of single foods and controlling the time interval between repeated exposures to the same food. Therefore, you will not eat too much of any given food at a single meal and you must diversify the selection of foods in your diet enough so that you will not eat members of the same food family at intervals that are too short. Controlling these factors will prevent single-food overdoses and the development of cumulative food reactions. You will find that your menus will become much more interesting as time goes by.

Don't worry. All this may sound complicated now, but with the training you will have given yourself during the Diagnostic Rotary Diet, and with a little more experience working with the Lifetime Arthritis Relief System, it will soon become second nature for you to plan and modify your diet as circumstances require. You will hardly need to think twice about what family a given food is part of. And very soon you will automatically remember what you ate and when you ate it last without referring to your diet schedule.

If you have a fixed allergy to one specific food or to several members of the same food family, you will avoid them altogether until you decide to treat them with professional help. You will quickly learn what mixed food products cause problems because they contain your offenders as "hidden" allergens. Begin by studying the list of hidden allergens on page 233, and develop the necessary habit of carefully reading the labels on all packaged food products that you may occasionally eat.

In general, if you find yourself craving certain foods, you must avoid them and distract yourself for as long as it takes for the craving to disappear. Divert yourself by activities other than eating; exercise is an excellent release. Recall as vividly as possible the pain that your recently controlled arthritis gave you in the past, and remember that this food you crave probably was one that caused it. Occasionally you may require some of the treatments or measures listed on pages 149–150 to block the craving and any other associated withdrawal symptoms you may be having.

A chemically susceptible person may develop an intense craving for a particular food—a former addictant—if he or she is exposed to and "turned on" by tobacco smoke, paint, mothballs, and the like. A food-allergic individual who is also allergic to certain molds or pollens may experience cravings for some addictive food after inhaling and absorbing the airborne allergens he or she reacts to.

On two occasions one of my depressed patients in Norwalk, Connecticut, who had many forms of allergic disorders became extremely hungry after contact with two of the many chemical offenders she was susceptible to. Accidental exposure to her husband's cigar smoke and to fresh paint "ignited" an uncontrollable craving for two of her major offenders—wheat and yeast (in bakery goods)—as well as an increased desire for baked goods in general. When she was reacting she satisfied her cravings with two extralarge Danish pastries or two large pieces of cake.

Other allergic patients reacting to the ingestion of one of their food offenders may have an overwhelming thirst, which can be satisfied by taking any kind of liquid, but in some cases allergic individuals are not satisfied unless they drink the specific addicting liquid substance, such as milk, apple juice, or orange juice, that they are experiencing withdrawal from. Another very interesting food-related observation I have made is that, during a reaction to certain foods a person is allergic to, the person will suddenly smell or taste the dust or mold (mildew)—inhalant allergens—that he or she is also sensitive to.

A major advantage of the Lifetime Rotary Diet is that in addition to controlling your allergic arthritis and other forms of internal or systemic allergies, it prevents potential allergens from becoming active causes of illness due to a cumulative allergen buildup in your system.

Hidden Allergens

Corn

aspirin
bacon
baking mixes
baking powder
beer
bleached flours
carbonated beverages
chewing gum
cough syrups
"Cream of" . . .
   cereals
glue on back of stamps
   and envelopes
gravies
instant coffee
instant teas
salad dressings

talcums
toothpaste
vanilla
vitamins

Dust

wine

Brewer's Yeast

B vitamins
beer
wine

Chlorine

anything with city
   water

coffee
juices
soda
tea
water

Antibiotics

beef
chicken
eggs
seafood (Fish markets
   and grocery stores
   treat their ice with
   antibiotics.)
turkey

Food Colorings	Baker's Yeast	malted products
butter	barbecue sauce	mayonnaise
certain fruits (e.g.,	brandy	mushrooms
oranges)	buttermilk	olives
fruit juices	catsup	pickles
margarine	cheese	rum
mouthwash	citrus fruit juices,	sauerkraut
processed meats	frozen or canned	vinegar
soft drinks	cottage cheese	vodka
toothpaste	gin	whiskey
	horseradish	wine
	leavening	

Rotation of potential offenders will prevent the development of active allergies to these substances. Therefore it is essential that you pay careful attention to your overall diet, and when you suddenly realize that you may be playing Russian roulette by eating too much of a given food, cut back! Diversifying and rotating your menus will benefit your entire state of health in many ways, including positive effects on the disorder in those arthritic joints and muscles that once were so sore and stiff.

Remember that adherence to the Lifetime Arthritis-Relief Rotary Diet, along with careful attention to environmental offenders, brings long-term arthritis relief in over eighty percent of all cases. *Its success is up to you.* Or, as stated by my brilliant and highly respected friend Dr. George Kroker, who has had remarkable successes in his La Crosse, Wisconsin, practice, "It takes patient compliance and follow-through to sustain improvement in arthritis." The absolutely necessary follow-through that can keep your joints pain-free and limber is entirely in your hands. You alone can keep yourself well, often without any drugs and in most cases without surgery; without the crippling misery of uncontrolled arthritis.

And what if your allergic arthritis is caused in whole or in part by environmental substances? The same principles apply as for food allergies. Keep your contact with all those chemicals and all other potential offenders below your allergic threshold. Although, as I noted in Chapter 9, it is often much more difficult to eliminate offending chemicals than offending foods, it is often possible to control their effects to a significant degree. But as I've also said, you can search for and find the substances to which you have proved yourself allergic or chemically susceptible and make many eliminations.

As the following checklist will remind you, dietary and environmental allergies are interrelated because of the allergic-threshold and total-allergic-load (burden) concepts. Just as you can tolerate well-spaced, small to moderate amounts of food that once brought you arthritic agony, you can live with a certain degree of exposure to airborne allergens and environmental chemical pollutants, contaminants, and additives—if you keep the total amount of all of them below the level at which you become reactive. By always being very careful to avoid or greatly limit the ingestion of foods to which you are allergic; by doing everything that you can to surround yourself with home, work, and daily activity environments that are as free as possible of pollutants; and by avoiding airborne allergens, you may be able to prevent the return of your arthritis pain permanently—or keep it very much under control.

Lifetime Arthritis-Prevention Checklist*

Dietary

Avoid all foods to which you have learned you have a fixed allergy (those that you have learned will flare up your arthritis, no matter what), but every six months or so try them again in a feeding test to see if you may have regained your tolerance.

As much as possible, drink bottled-in-glass spring water.† Eat foods uncontaminated by chemical preservatives or other processing agents. Buy natural, organically grown foods when you can, and cook in glass, stainless steel or ceramic pottery.

Avoid foods for which you feel a craving; substitute other foods or activities.

Environmental

As far as possible, remove every one of those substances from your home and work environments that you have proven will flare up your arthritis.

Remove (or prevent contact with) from your daily environment as many as possible of the chemically active substances that may not bother you yet but that are potentially hazardous, such as tobacco smoke, petroleum-based products, and common household chemicals like detergents, disinfectants, insect sprays, chlorine, etc.

Continue to use natural products for domestic and personal cleaning and your clothing.

Should your immediate environ-

---

*By following these simple guidelines, it is very likely that you can prevent many arthritis flare-ups, because you will keep your exposure to all known and probable arthritis-inducing substances below your threshold level.

†At the very least, remove the chlorine from your tap water by boiling it for ten minutes or by using a charcoal filter that may be connected to the faucet. Be sure to change the cartridge in the filter at proper intervals. One teaspoon of sodium thiosulfate from your pharmacy will remove the chlorine from a bathtub full of tap water. Do not use this substance in drinking or cooking water.

11

Nutrition and Arthritis*

Once you have eliminated or greatly reduced the severity of your allergic-arthritis symptoms by forming the habit of eating tolerated amounts of "safe" foods in rotation and controlling the chemical pollutants and inhalants in your environment, you will feel much better in general. The higher your overall level of health, of course, the better you'll feel. Also, we have found that the better the general health of a person, the higher the "allergic resistance" and the lower the susceptibility to active and potential allergens.

An excellent way to maintain yourself at the peak of health is to provide yourself with the best nutrition. As the Arthritis Foundation has stated, "Good nutrition is essential for good health whether you have arthritis or not; and it is even more important when your body must resist and fight off the ravages of a disease like arthritis."

I fully agree with this statment. But, unfortunately, the Arthritis Foundation has completely rejected the nondrug nutritional therapy that has evolved from biochemical-nutritional research on arthritis. The role of specific nutrients is not merely ignored in the foundation's official "authoritative" statements on the treatment of arthritis; the use of specific nutrients is condemned despite published

*This chapter was written with the assistance of Elaine Fox, Ph.D., director of the Division of Nutritional Medicine, North Nassau Mental Health Center, Manhasset, Long Island. We also received the cooperation of doctors Ellis, Horrobin, Kaufman, and Reich, for which we thank them.

clinical and laboratory reports of demonstrable improvement in arthritis after proper treatment by nutritional supplementation. It seems to me that the foundation's interest in drug research has led to an unbalanced overall view in this area.

Nutrition plays a dual role in the patient who is suffering from arthritis. There are a number of nutritional therapies that have been reported to have helped thousands of arthritics. When they are combined with a course of hyposensitizing injections of allergenic extracts and the removal of the environmental factors that can precipitate arthritis, nutritional supplements often provide additional help. Nutritional support of the allergic individual may reduce the impact of the allergen on the patient and decrease the intensity of the arthritic as well as other coexisting allergies. In some cases nutritional treatment has actually blocked the negative, arthritis-evoking allergic response. By removing the environmental substances that are causing the arthritis and supporting the patient internally by means of superior nutrition, we have a greater likelihood of achieving even more relief.

A number of vitamins and minerals can help the allergic sufferer react less severely after exposure to an offending substance. Vitamin C and pantothenic acid have been shown to be natural antihistamines. Histamine is one of the mischief makers that are released during an allergic reaction, and anything that functions as a natural antihistamine may be helpful.

It has been demonstrated that allergic individuals have an increased need for Vitamin C, and it has also been found that abnormally small amounts of vitamin C are present in their blood. Not only is vitamin C an antihistamine, it is necessary for proper functioning of the adrenal glands, which produce hormones that help combat allergic reactions. For the arthritic who is taking aspirin, a supplement of vitamin C is necessary, since aspirin depletes this vitamin. In fact, Dr. William Kaufman has found some cases of arthritis that were actually caused by aspirin.

Pantothenic acid also supports the function of the adrenal glands. British physicians E. C. Barton-Wright and W. A. Eliot observed that the blood levels of pantothenic acid were low in rheumatoid arthritics, and some of these people were definitely helped by a supplement of pantothenic acid; fresh royal jelly given along with pantothenic acid was even more effective.* (Royal jelly is the richest natural source of pantothenic acid.)

*Lancet, October, 1963.

Our adrenal glands are two small organs located next to the upper ends of the kidneys that help us deal with stress. The severity of allergic reaction is often increased during stress, and anything that helps the allergic individual handle stress more effectively is important, such as filling the need of the adrenals for vitamin C and pantothenic acid in order to manufacture their stress-relieving hormones.

The permeability (penetrability) of cell walls is of vital importance in the allergic person, since an excessively permeable cell wall (membrane) allows unwanted substances that can cause reactions to enter the cell. A deficiency of protein in the diet can cause this undesirable condition. Any substance that decreases excessive cell wall permeability helps reduce symptoms by keeping illness-evoking agents out. Vitamin C and the bioflavinoids (nutritional factors found in nature along with vitamin C) also decrease cell-wall permeability. Bioflavinoids protect Vitamin C against oxidation (chemical breakdown), making the vitamin C more effective.

Vitamin E and the mineral selenium stabilize cell walls, and this is very important in treating allergies. Vitamin A decreases the permeability of cells in the skin and the mucous membranes. When large amounts of vitamins A and E were given to adults, their cells showed a rapid and marked increase in ability to prevent foreign substances from penetrating them. Calcium also reduces excessive permeability of cell membranes.

Vitamin-B complex, especially B_6 (pyridoxine), decreases allergic symptoms. When given together, large amounts of vitamin B_6 and C have actually blocked allergic reactions in some people.

Toxic minerals such as lead and mercury can interfere with optimum functioning of the body, and a chemical analysis of scalp hair can be performed to measure the level of these toxic minerals. An accurately performed trace-mineral analysis, properly interpreted, may yield clues to health problems, but the final word is not in on this matter. I believe that hair testing is being commercially exploited at present.

A number of researchers have indicated that many allergic people have problems in their digestive tracts. Some have obvious signs, such as constipation, diarrhea, bloating, distention, cramps, flatulence, belching, bad breath, and even pieces of undigested food in the stool, while others have no apparent gastrointestinal symptoms even though they have serious digestive malfunctions. Therefore, a simple discussion of the digestion process seems appropriate here.

The first phase, carbohydrate digestion, takes place in the mouth, where the enzyme-containing saliva begins the breakdown of starches as food is masticated and mixed with saliva. Digestion of protein starts in the stomach, and this process will not be efficient if there is inadequate production of hydrochloric acid by the acid-forming cells of the stomach.

Digestive enzymes and sodium bicarbonate from the pancreas are released into the small intestines to continue the protein digestion that began in the stomach, in addition to continuing the digestion of fats and carbohydrates. Although stomach acid is necessary to digest protein, the opposite medium (alkaline) is necessary for the pancreatic enzymes to work in the small intestine.

Two conditions influence whether there will be enough sodium bicarbonate produced by the pancreas for the proper functioning of the pancreatic enzymes: the amount of stomach acid and the supply of zinc. If there is not enough stomach acid, the pancreas will not be stimulated to produce enough bicarbonate ions, and the amount of acid present in the stomach has an influence on all digestion.

Betaine hydrochloride can be used to increase the amount of stomach acid. It is available in 5-grain tablets and can be taken immediately before a meal. Betaine is usually taken for only one or two months, and then the dose is gradually reduced and eliminated. In most cases the body has the ability to increase its own production of stomach acid if it is helped for a short period of time. Persons with an ulcer history should not experiment with hydrochloric-acid supplements. They require the advice of a physician.

In zinc deficiency, the pancreas cannot produce enough bicarbonate, and this makes pancreatic enzymes less active. A small zinc supplement may help people with digestive problems.

Sometimes bicarbonate is given with pancreatic enzymes, but this should be done with the advice of a knowledgeable health care practitioner, since the bicarbonate can neutralize the acid in the stomach and interfere with digestion rather than aid it.

Recent research indicates that pancreatic proteolytic enzymes (enzymes involved in protein digestion) serve another important function in the body. Some of these enzymes are absorbed directly into the blood and carried to areas of inflammation and directly reduce the inflammation.

Bromelain from the pineapple, papain from the papaya, aloe from the aloe vera plant, and garlic all have digestive properties whose use as supplements has been successfully demonstrated by William Philpott, M.D.

When the digestive system is malfunctioning and there is incomplete protein digestion, the body does not get the raw materials (the amino acids that are released by normal protein digestion) to build the proper enzymes. This becomes a vicious cycle; the enzymes are necessary for proper digestion, and if the body cannot manufacture enough of them, digestion will decrease, leading to fewer raw materials being available to the body. Supplementing with amino acids in the form of predigested protein or synthetic amino acids, the body can build the necessary machinery to carry out the digestive process. Remember that a sensitive individual can react to any of the digestive aids and should be cautious when first trying them.

Superoxide dysmutase is another enzyme that is helpful in the treatment of arthritis. It is effective in the control of inflammation. Until recently it was only available to physicians in the injectable form under the name orgotein. Although it may not be as effective when taken by mouth as in the injectable form, some patients have had remarkable results using as few as two or three tablets per day. The usual dose is higher.

William Kaufman, M.D., Ph.D., of Stratford, Connecticut, winner of the 1978 Tom Spies Memorial·Award in Nutrition, was the first physician to use niacinamide (vitamin B-3; niacin is another form of B_3), one of the B-complex vitamins, in the treatment of arthritis. His initial observations were made late in 1940. At that time Dr. Kaufman treated many patients who had developed a niacinamide deficiency less severe than classic pellagra. These patients had a wide range of nervous-system symptoms, widespread tissue swelling, weakness and excessive tiredness, stomach and intestinal complaints, and women often had inflamed vaginal tissues. Niacinamide treatment cleared up all these troubles promptly.

Dr. Kaufman also made an unexpected observation, something very important that had never been reported before. Patients who were given this vitamin—and also had arthritis—had great improvement in their ability to move their arthritic joints, and they had much less joint stiffness, discomfort, and pain.

To be certain that niacinamide was responsible for the improvements observed in their arthritis, without his patients' knowledge, Dr. Kaufman substituted an inert, look-alike tablet (a placebo) for the vitamin B_3 tablets. After seven to ten days without niacinamide, the arthritis was as bad as it had been before starting niacinamide treatment. Then, again without the patients' knowledge, he reintroduced the niacinamide treatment. All patients improved as dramatically as they had when they were first treated. Thus, with scientific objectivity, Dr. Kaufman proved that niacinamide was responsible for all the improvements that he and the arthritic patients observed.

After bread and cereal products were vitamin-enriched in 1943, few patients had the broad range of symptoms previously described. But many, including those with obvious arthritis, had impaired joint mobility that was improved by niacinamide treatment.

In 1943 Dr. Kaufman developed or adapted a series of instruments to measure joint movement with scientific precision. He measured the range of movement of twenty specific joints and developed his Joint Range Index (JRI). This single number diagnosed the patient's joint status as follows:

JRI RATING	JOINT STATUS
96 to 100	no joint dysfunction
86 to 95	slight joint dysfunction
71 to 85	moderate joint dysfunction
56 to 70	severe joint dysfunction
55 or less	extremely severe joint dysfunction

Since wear and tear of joints gradually exceeds the body's capacity to repair them as the person ages, the JRI technique detected ongoing joint deterioration years before osteoarthritis could be diagnosed. Most patients with moderate joint dysfunction and all patients with severe or extremely severe joint dysfunction had corresponding grades of severity of diagnosable osteoarthritis.

After measuring a patient's JRI, Dr. Kaufman selected a suitable starting schedule of niacinamide treatment for that individual. An acceptable response to therapy was a rise of 6 to 12 JRI units the first month and 1/2 to 1 JRI units each month thereafter.) Sometimes the niacinamide dosage schedule had to be adjusted upward to get the desired degree of improvement. Eventually the patient's improvement in joint mobility would stabilize at the highest possible level, taking into consideration the amount of wear and tear on his or her joints resulting from ordinary physical activities.

The dosage schedule that provided satisfactory rates of improvement was used for continuous maintenance therapy. Improvement in joint mobility was sustained as the patient took niacinamide as prescribed, continued to eat a diet adequate in calories and protein, and did not subject joints to overuse or injury.

Dr. Kaufman found that joints so severely damaged by arthritis as to indicate end-of-the-road deterioration are very unlikely to show appreciable increases in joint mobility or other benefits in response to niacinamide therapy. He also noted that adding other vitamins to niacinamide therapy did not speed the rate of recovery from impaired joint mobility. However, these might provide other health benefits.

Dr. Kaufman emphasized that his niacinamide treatment for therapy of joint dysfunction should *not* be used for self-treatment but should always be supervised by a physician.

From 1944 until he stopped practicing in 1964, he usually prescribed from 900 to 4000 milligrams of niacinamide a day in four to twelve or more divided doses. The specific dose level and schedule of niacinamide intake was based on each patient's initial JRI. No single dose ever exceeded 250 milligrams. Used in this manner, Dr. Kaufman's vitamin-B_3 therapy was well tolerated and generally effective in improving joint function. As JRI measurements improved, his patients noted increased joint mobility; greater freedom in the use of joints; decreased joint stiffness, discomfort and pain; less fatiguability; and an improved sense of well-being.

Two complications could cause a temporary or more sustained setback: joint injury, including that caused by excess muscle tension and overuse of joints; and the onset of allergic arthritis in susceptible persons whose allergic overload must be corrected by various ecologic techniques that accomplish what the antiallergic properties of niacinamide cannot completely control. Each of these conditions required separate treatment, during which niacinamide therapy was always continued at the optimal level.

Dr. John Ellis of Mt. Pleasant, Texas, has pioneered the use of vitamin B_6 (pyridoxine) in the treatment of arthritis and in carpal-tunnel syndrome (swelling and/or numbness of the hand due to a compression or irritation of a nerve that passes through the wrist). Dr. Ellis found that vitamin-B_6 deficiency causes swelling of synovial tissue in joints and tendons. When the synovia lining the joints of fingers, elbows, shoulders, hips, knees, ankles, and toes are inflamed, this is referred to as arthritis.

Using 150 milligrams of B_6 daily (Dr. Ellis told me he prefers that patients take 50 milligrams three times a day, but if they are going to forget to do so they should take the entire 150 milligrams in the morning), the following improvements were noted: (1) reduction of swelling in hands and fingers, (2) improved range of finger flexion, (3) reduction of tenderness and pain in finger joints, (4) improved coordination of finger movements, (5) elimination of numbness and tingling in hands and fingers, (6) prevention of transient paralysis of the arms at night, (7) halting of leg cramps and muscle spasms at night, (8) reduction or elimination of shoulder pain, (9) improvement of shoulder and arm function.

In cases of carpal-tunnel syndrome, every one of Dr. Ellis's patients improved upon taking B_6 for twelve weeks in 150-milligram (50 milligram three times a day) doses.

According to Dr. Ellis, there are millions of Americans who have clinical vitamin B_6 deficiencies, who have been diagnosed as having a large number of diseases, including arthritis.

The treatment of arthritis with vitamins A and D and the minerals present in bone meal has been championed by my friend Carl Reich, M.D., a Canadian physician. Carl views arthritis as a stress-related disease that occurs in individuals who are unable to handle biologic stresses. Using megadoses of vitamins A and D and mineral-rich bone meal, a much larger percentage of patients experienced relief from pain, swelling, and disability than could be expected from conventional drug therapy. A note of caution: vitamins A and D are fat soluble and they are stored in the liver. Doses greater than 25,000 International Units (IVs) of vitamin A and 1,000 IVs of vitamin D should be supervised by a professional health care practitioner who is nutritionally oriented.

Vitamins A and D are found in large amounts in cod-liver oil, which is reported to have helped many arthritics. Along with a modification of diet, nutrition writer Dale Alexander suggests taking one tablespoon of emulsified cod-liver oil in fresh orange juice or milk on an empty stomach at least three or four hours after the evening meal or one or two hours before breakfast.

Researchers have shown vitamin E, vitamin C, vitamin-B complex, and the minerals zinc and magnesium to be helpful in the treatment of arthritis, and there has been considerable speculation regarding the mechanisms by which these vitamins and minerals accomplish this feat. Recently the probable method of action of these nutrients in relieving the symptoms of arthritis has been elucidated. David Horrobin, M.D., Ph.D., a noted authority on prostaglandins, has kindly supplied us with information concerning research on their role in arthritis.

Prostaglandins are hormonelike substances that help control the function of every organ in the body; they can influence susceptibility to infection and inflammation. Prostaglandins are formed from essential fatty acids (essential since we must have them and they cannot be made by our own body), which must come from sources in the diet.

An excess of one type of prostaglandin, called E 2, and an

inadequate production of the E 1 type are associated with inflammatory states. The excess of the E 2 series of prostaglandins seems responsible for much of the local damage, while the inadequacy of the E 1 series of prostaglandins contributes to the immune deficits in many inflammatory states. The prostaglandin E 1 blocks responses to the substances like histamine that cause inflammation in the body, and therefore it is desirable to increase the body's production of this beneficial substance.

Formation of prostaglandin E 1 requires linoleic acid, an essential fatty acid found in large quantities in vegetable oils and organ meats. Linoleic acid is converted to prostaglandins through a number of complicated biochemical processes that need not be discussed here. To become biologically active, linoleic acid must be converted to gamma-linolenic acid. Processing of vegetable oils to solid cooking fats and margarines may convert much of the natural and nutritionally valuable linoleic acid to a form that does not have essential fatty acid activity but actually acts as an antiessential fatty acid.

The formation of prostaglandin E 1 from linoleic acid requires magnesium, zinc, and vitamins B_3, B_6, and C; a deficiency of any one of these could interfere with the production of prostaglandin E 1. These are the vitamins and minerals that have been successful in the treatment of arthritis. In people whose gamma-linolenic-acid formation is reduced, prostaglandin-E 1 production may be restored by giving gamma-linolenic acid directly, and the only readily available sources of gamma-linolenic acid are human milk and evening primrose oil. Moderate to high alcohol intake, diabetes, aging, cancer, and viral infections are factors that block the conversion of linoleic acid to gamma-linolenic acid.

The E 2 series of prostaglandins that cause local damage arise from arachidonic acid, which is found in meat, some diary products, and some seaweeds. One of the diets that has been used in the treatment of arthritis and has helped thousands of individuals suffering from inflammation and painful joints removes most of these foods.

Collin H. Dong, M.D., found that many foods high in fat, such as meat and dairy products, were contributing to his severe arthritic condition. He developed a diet drastically lower in saturated-fat content, which is more like the typical Oriental diet than the typical Western diet. He excludes: (1) meat in any form, including broth; (2) fruit of any kind, including tomatoes; (3) dairy products, including egg yolks, cheese, and yogurt; (4) vinegar or any other acid; (5) pepper of any variety; (6) hot spices; (7) chocolate; (8) dry-roasted nuts; (9) alcoholic beverages, particularly wine; (10) soft drinks; and (11) all additives, preservatives, and chemicals, especially monosodium glutamate. His diet has been successful for thousands of arthritis sufferers.

I do not know if Dr. Dong's diet works by influencing the balance of prostaglandins, but this certainly is possible and may be an important factor in some cases. My clinical experience strongly suggests that Dr. Dong's diet is effective because it eliminates many allergenic foods and biologically active chemical agents that cause joint and muscle reactions in a large number of people who have arthritis. I believe that in some cases arthritis is probably a reaction to both.

It is interesting to note that Dr. Dong has excluded tomatoes and peppers from the diet of individuals suffering from arthritis, since another popular diet that has helped a large number of people also excludes these foods. Norman Childers, professor of horticulture at Rutgers, the State University of New Jersey, discovered that the group of plants called the nightshades can cause symptoms of arthritis in sensitive people. Dr. Childers was inspired to try a nightshade-avoidance diet to relieve his painful arthritis because he realized that livestock that grazed on the solanine-containing nightshade weeds often develop such painful joints that they are sometimes found kneeling, because standing is too painful.

The nightshades include the white potato (not the yam or sweet potato); tomato; eggplant; peppers, including pimento, paprika, cayenne, and chili (but excluding black and white pepper), and tobacco. It may be hard for you to believe that these commonly eaten foods can cause a problem so severe as to incapacitate arthritis-prone individuals, but I have repeatedly demonstrated that any food has the potential to cause severe reactions in allergically sensitive individuals. In the case of the nightshade-family foods, some of the problem may be that of solanine toxicity rather than allergy, but I have produced acute arthritis flare-ups with just a few drops of dilute extracts of potato, tomato, green pepper, and eggplant, clearly showing that a high degree of sensitivity is present because of the minute quanitities employed (and there can be very little solanine in a few drops of my testing solutions. Solanine, a chemical common to all these plants, has been shown to interfere with acetylcholine metabolism, which is vital to muscle function, and this may be one of the modes of action in causing trouble).

Corresponding with thousands of arthritics who volunteered to follow his diet, Dr. Childers found that 70 percent experienced some degree of relief after avoiding the nightshade vegetables, from mild to dramatic.* For many the improvement did not come for at least three months; for some it took as long as an entire year of avoidance before they experienced a great deal of improvement. In general, the younger you are, the less time it takes to see improvement. If you do want to try the no-nightshade diet, it is important to read labels, since there are a large number of canned and processed foods to which at least one of the nightshades has been added. Dr. Childers has also found that a large number of people are sensitive to artificial sweeteners and should avoid them as well. Here we are dealing with a coal-tar-derived chemical agent, saccharin, that has provoked thousands of physical and mental reactions in my office.

During the late 1960s and early 1970s, a research project was developed to screen different types of shellfish from around the world in the search for a possible treatment for cancer. As a result of this project, a substance from the New Zealand green lipid mussel was found to be beneficial for many people suffering from arthritis. An extract of this New Zealand green lippid mussel is now available and has helped approximately 60 percent of those who have used it for the relief of arthritic symptoms.

It takes approximately three weeks from the time of starting treatment for the first signs of a beneficial reaction to be noticed, although some people respond as rapidly as in one week while others may not notice a change in their condition for as long as fifteen weeks. Neither the age of the person nor the duration of the illness can be used to predict how long it will take to start feeling any benefit. It is important to point out that some people get worse temporarily before getting better. They may experience a flare-up of symptoms, such as an increase in pain and stiffness.

In addition to relief of symptoms, many patients report a feeling of well-being. It is not clear how the extract of the green lippid mussel works, and all the efforts to isolate and test various components of the extract have not been successful as of this writing. For further information see *Relief from Arthritis,* by John C. Croft (Wellingborough, Australia: Thorsons Publishers, Ltd., 1979).

The purpose of the information in this chapter is to offer as much help as is available to every person who is suffering from arthritis. It may not be possible for you to identify all the dietary and environmental factors that are causing your arthritis. If you can discover the

---

*There are so many food-intolerant people among the millions of cases of arthritis that it is possible to find thousands of people with any kind of allergy that one is looking for.

most significant and treat or remove those, and then, using nutrition, reduce the impact of the environment on yourself, this can offer a great deal of relief. It is important to remember that disease is an interaction between the individual and his or her environment.

In discussing this interaction, J. M. May used an analogy that is worth quoting. "It is as though I had on a table three dolls—one of glass, another of celluloid, and a third of steel—and I chose to hit the three dolls with a hammer, using equal strength. The first doll would break, the second would scar and the third would emit a pleasant musical sound."* If we think of you as the doll and the hammer as the environment, nutrition can possibly change you from a glass doll to a celluloid or plastic doll. If you are a doll of steel, then you are among the lucky ones who do not react to either foods or the environment with symptoms of arthritis or any of the numerous physical and/or mental-emotional disorders that affect millions of our fellow humans who are allergy-prone or susceptible to the chemical environment.

*J. M. May, *Annals of New York Academy of Science* 84 (1960): 789–94.

12

Finding Help—Doctors' Attitudes— Laboratory Tests

How do you feel? How did we make out with your arthritis? Are things a little better? Were you definitely helped but for just a while? Has there been a moderate improvement? Are you completely free of your symptoms or very much better? Did you clear up and then "lose it"? Are you happy with the results of our "joint" efforts? Did you learn enough from personal experience to feel optimistic—to feel hopeful—even though the results to date have not met your expectations?

I know that those of you who now know how it feels not to have arthritis will have little trouble in carefully following my Lifetime Arthritis Relief System. You have an effective self-help program that really works for you.

Not all readers who can be helped will have had the degree of success they looked forward to when they acquired my book. If you are among them, you can still make another big step toward bringing your arthritis under control.

If your questionnaire responses and/or your testing experiences indicate that you are a victim of allegic arthritis, but you have not been able to pinpoint and do something about the as-yet-unidentified major allergens in your case or have not found significant relief in the program you have developed and, followed . . .

If you feel you have managed to eliminate some but not all the allergens from your diet or environment because you can't remodel or move away, change jobs, or give up your hobby or your pets . . .

If you know that you have determined some or many of your arthritis-causing sensitivities but have not been able to eliminate enough of them to feel as well as you believe you can . . .

If your reactions to some of the tests have been quite severe and yet something isn't working right . . .

If your allergic threshold for experiencing symptoms is very low . . .

Then you would do well to consult with a clinical ecologist. The names of some of them have already been mentioned in the preceding pages, and you will find a list of some of the others and clinics at the end of this chapter. You can also write to my friend Del Stigler, M.D., the secretary of the Society for Clinical Ecology. His address is noted on page 257. Request the names of the qualified physicians in your area. Be sure to include a self-addressed and stamped envelope.

You may ask your personal physician for a letter of referral to an ecologist, but this is not at all necessary because you can make your own appointment directly. You do not have to bring all your records with you, and it is possible that you may have difficulty getting them if your doctor does not go along with your idea. You can demand them through your local, county, or state medical society, or through a phone call or note from your lawyer if you wish. I want to emphasize the fact that the most important information in the majority of cases, including yours, is filed away in your memory, reflected in your eating habits, or may be found in your home and work environment, life-style, and so on—an important part of the answer to your problem is right at your fingertips.

In some instances it is possible that you will not get much encouragement from your doctor. It is an unfortunate fact that many physicians still remain unaware of the clinical effectiveness of the bioecologic approach to arthritis and many other serious ailments, and they frequently attempt to dissuade patients from trying it. This tragic situation occurred in my practice when I treated an allergic-arthritis patient several years ago. Her doctor refused to believe that I had performed reproducible arthritis-provoking tests, even though some single-blind tests were repeated two or three times to be sure, and he ignored the demonstrated effectiveness of my treatment. Something very good—something important—had happened to a patient whose illness he could not control. He could not bring himself, for whatever reason, to investigate the matter personally by a phone call or visit with me, even though his patient was better. As a professional healer, he had no understanding of why she was better. Instead of welcoming the good news, he resisted it—fought it emotionally. And instead of taking advantage of my standing invitation for any licensed physician to avail himself of my open-door visiting policy, he chose to ignore my offer to share and teach. My open door is there for any professionals and students involved in the healing arts (as well as educators and other individuals with a legitimate interest in my work).

With the patients' permission and in a manner that does not interfere with my office routine, testing may be observed and the welcome visitor may sit in and to a limited extent (within the bounds of common sense and professional comportment) actually participate in consultations. To this day I thank Ted Randolph for the many hours and opportunities he generously gave me almost twenty years ago.

I established my visiting policy to educate my colleagues in the true spirit of Hippocrates—to repay those respected teachers and colleagues (and very cooperative, caring patients) from whom I have learned, by passing on to others the invaluable knowledge and skills that I have acquired. For years I have offered my professional brothers a golden opportunity to receive invaluable and indispensable clinical information that can be employed immediately for the benefit of the hundreds of thousands of patients who come to them with hope and trust.

And, sadly, because of emotionally generated close-mindedness, this unreasonable situation still persists and is responsible for the long-distance trips of increasing numbers of disappointed and misdiagnosed patients who eventually find their way to one of the environmentally controlled, hospital-based ecologic units. Each of these essential facilities is under the direction of an ecologist who has the good fortune to have a forward-looking administrator or board of trustees in their local hospital.

In late 1981 I successfully treated a patient who had been crippled by arthritis for ten years; she had traveled a considerable distance to come to my office, over the objections of a rheumatologist, who had tried every drug available on her and then told her there was no hope. But there *is* hope! Very real hope for eight hundred out of every thousand of you if you work hard at it, and for another hundred of you if you will enter an environmentally controlled ecologic unit and let one of my colleagues help you. Even if you have had only limited success after following the techniques described in this book, the odds are in your favor that you will find more relief with the help of an ecologically oriented physician.

Remember, it is a matter of official hospital records that Ted Randolph in Illinois, Bill Rea in Texas, and Murray Carroll and Thurman Bullock in North Carolina (with the indispensable contributions of their hardworking associates) did a three-hospital cooperative study on rheumatoid arthritis and independently established the causative role of dietary and environmental factors in this devastating illness.

And my own double-blind study, for which I again thank Tony Conte for his efforts and generous cooperation, also showed the importance of the same identifiable and controllable agents. I also wish to remind you that ecologically oriented colleagues here and abroad have made the same observations. *Don't give up until you have done your very best to prove that you cannot be helped.*

When you seek the assistance of one of these physicians, what can you expect?

Diagnostic techniques and methods of treatment will vary to some extent from office to office, but the fundamental concepts will be those shared with the Alan Mandell Center for Bio-Ecologic Diseases. A qualified clinical ecologist will:

> Conduct his or her professional activities in an office, clinic, or hospital setting, having taken measures to have a suitable physical environment that is as free as possible of chemicals, dust, molds, pollens, and other indoor air pollutants.
>
> Require from each potential patient a personal chronological report of his or her lifetime health history from birth to current medical problems, and a list of medications used and responses to them.
>
> Use detailed questionnaires and interviews in depth with the ecologist and members of the professional staff to focus on the ecologically significant aspects of what is usually a multiple-system, multiple-symptom disorder, and look for information that suggests the most likely environmental and dietary factors in each case.

Spend at least several days and up to two weeks carefully testing for sensitivity to a comprehensive group of environmental allergens, using various solutions and inhalation tests.

Perform a simple but very important (when indicated) neurological examination for "soft signs" of minor nervous system injury and dysfunction relating to development and cerebral hemispheric dominance.

This may be done on an outpatient basis, as I do with 95 to 97 percent of my patients, or in very severe and complex cases, by hospitalizing patients for a period of therapeutic fasting and testing in the controlled environment of an ecologic unit. At the Alan Mandell Center we first have patients complete our questionnaire if they have not done so at home and then mailed it to us; and then we either have our initial consultation or begin a series of sublingual provocation tests, followed later that day by the initial consultation.

Although different specialists may use different techniques, the technicians on my professional staff conduct our symptom-duplicating tests by placing a few drops of allergenic extracts of foods, molds, pollens, dust, and the like, and solutions of various chemical substances, under the patient's tongue in a carefully programmed sequence involving different strengths of these known environmental offenders. There are other techniques in use, but this is the one I have found to be very effective and I employ it almost exclusively, along with nasal inhalation challenges with natural airborne allergens in their native state.

As each test is performed, the patient and his or her technician observe and record all the details of signs and symptoms that develop as the patient reacts. During testing, we also assess the patient's balance, vision, walking, reading, speech, and penmanship, and the like as indicated. Penmanship samples are saved for future use, and video documentation is also employed when indicated. In addition, the clinical ecologist will:

Retest when this is indicated and then reintroduce the test-identified allergens in their usual form to observe directly the patient's responses for confirmation of laboratory findings and for patient education.

Treat the allergic-ecologic disorder by prescribing a diet, resistance-building nutritional supplements, and a program of environmental modifications that reduces exposure or, hopefully, eliminates the offending allergens and environmental incitants from the patient's life. Many cases will require an allergic desensitization program (immunotherapy) that consists of the administration, by injection or sublingually (under the tongue), of allergenic extracts of substances that will eventually control an allergy unless there is massive exposure that overwhelms the allergic individual's defenses.

Provide a follow-up service for continuing reporting, consultation, and advice that is absolutely necessary as a case progresses and various developments occur.

Cytotoxic, RAST, and Hair Mineral Tests

I do not and will not employ cytotoxic testing, which is very convenient but not nearly as accurate a diagnostic technique. Technicians studying the same test material in the same laboratory disagree with each other in their interpretation of such tests. It is most unfortunate that cytotoxic testing has been adopted by some physicians seeking shortcuts. Cytotoxic testing is also used by a group of untrained individuals who are not knowledgeable in the area of dietary ecologic analysis and treatment of illness. In my opinion, they should not be permitted to mislead the public or to charge for services in which they have no expertise. This is a complex and extremely important health area, not for amateurs, since food allergy profoundly affects the physical and mental health of the unsuspecting clients they are unprepared to give comprehensive treatment to.

The constuction of diagnostic and therapeutic diets requires extensive knowledge of the many facets of food allergy and food intolerance as well as an adequate medical background. Any individual who lacks this expertise is unqualified to prescribe diets or to counsel sick individuals by using the information obtained from this overworked and abused blood test (that does have definite academic interest but should remain as a research tool at present).

The RAST test, a technique I discarded many years ago because it is of so little value in food allergy, is scientifically attractive and carries an intriguing air of mystery since some radioactive materials are employed in its performance. However, it is no more accurate than a skin test, which has an 80 percent error factor in diagnosing food allergy, and it costs at least two to four times as much per test as a conventional skin test.

I know some gadget-minded physicians have bought the special and expensive electronic equipment that is required to do RAST testing in their own offices. And there are other physicians who also become involved because they see themselves as modern doctors keeping up with the latest developments, even though the answers they get from their equipment are not one bit more useful to their patients than the economical but only 20 percent accurate skin tests for food allergy.

Hair analysis to assess a patient's nutritional state is at present an income-producing, commercialized laboratory procedure that probably has some merit. For the most part, the value of this test remains to be clearly demonstrated. The idea is attracive, but to date, the laboratories do not agree with each other in a number of areas and their results are not always comparable. For example, a high level of a particular mineral may be interpreted as an excess in the body or as an indication that the body is losing that mineral into the hair and is deficient.

Many thousands of people have found relief from their arthritis and other serious internal allergies through these proven medical techniques that are directed at the specific cause of the disorders. If by reading this book you have come to realize that your arthritis (or the arthritis of someone to whom you are close) is an allergic-ecologic condition, but you have not been able to find complete relief by following my system on your own, I urge you to consult with one of the qualified professionals whose valuable services are available to you.

This is a partial list of individuals and organizations that can provide additional information concerning allergies (including chemical intolerances), clinical ecology, and related areas.

Chemically sensitive individuals qualify (with a doctor's verification) for "Talking Books" for the blind, a free service. Contact your local library or: Library of Congress, National Library Services for the Blind and Handicapped, Washington, D.C., 20542, 1-800-424-9100, toll free.

Associations, Support Groups, and Their Publications
(When requesting information, if possible ʌnclose a stamped, self-addressed envelope.)

Action Against Allergy (AAA)
43 The Downs
London, England SW20 8HG
(01) 947-5082

> Provides personal information by mail or phone, sponsors a lending library, lectures, films, and book services on clinical ecology. Provides a list of physicians and locations. Write or call for additional information.

The Human Ecology Action League (HEAL)
505 N. Lakeshore Drive
Suite 6506
Chicago, Illinois 60611
(312) 836-0422

> An organization that represents the aims and programs of patients, physicians and others interested in environmental health. Publishes a national newsletter. Write or call for additional information. Donations are welcomed.

Human Ecology Foundation of Canada
R.R. #1, Goodwood
Ontario, Canada LOC 1AO

> Quarterly newsletter is available

The Human Ecology Research Foundation
505 N. Lake Shore Drive
Chicago, Illinois, 60611
(312) 828-9481

> Supports medical research, application, and publication in the field of human ecology; source for reprints of Dr. Theron G. Randolph's numerous articles describing the relationships between chronic physical and mental illnesses, food, drugs, and chemicals in the environment.

Human Ecology Research Foundation of the Southwest, Inc.
12110 Webb Chapel Road, Suite 305E
Dallas, Texas 75234
(214) 620-0620

> The above foundation is a National Information and Referral Center.

> It was formed in 1975 as a nonprofit corporation. Its purpose is to study the effect of the environment on the body's basic biochemistry. A program has been devised to demonstrate an acute cause-and-effect relationship between these two factors.

> Ecologically oriented materials are available for reproduction through the Human Ecology Research Library. Publications and products designed especially for the chemically sensitive, information on environmentally designed housing and other related items are available. Donations are accepted and encouraged to continue further research to help find a cure for ecologic disease. The foundation is a source for reprints of articles and publications of Dr. William Rea's research.

Also available for purchase is *Guidelines,* a comprehensive resource guide to facilitate the finding of safe products and resources for the chemically sensitive patient. Mail-order shops as well as other sources from around the country have been used. It provides information for such areas as air conditioners, filters, purifiers, appliances, automotives, bedding, publications, building materials, dental care, travel and much more.

Contact the foundation for price and availability of *Guidelines— A Compilation of Products and Resources for the Chemically Sensitive.* by Alice Billman.

Alan Mandell Center for Bio-Ecologic Diseases
3 Brush Street
Norwalk, Connecticut 06850
(203) 838-4706

An organization devoted to research, education, and treatment of ecologic diseases. Has reprinted papers by Dr. Marshall Mandell. Write for information.

New England Foundation for Allergic and Environmental Diseases
3 Brush Street
Norwalk, Connecticut 06850

A nonprofit, tax-free organization devoted to research, dissemination of information, and treatment of allergic and environmental diseases. Donations are welcomed.

Society for Clinical Ecology
Del Stigler, M.D., Secretary
2005 Franklin St., #409
Denver, Colorado 80205
(303) 831-7335

A society of physicians, scientists, and other professionals dedicated to the investigation of chemical susceptibility and allergies. Holds meetings, conducts basic and advanced seminars, and publishes archives. *The Society can provide names of clinical ecologists in various parts of the United States and abroad.*

Environmental Control Centers and Isolated Rooms

The following is a partial list of environmental control centers and physicians employing comprehensive environmental control in isolated rooms.

Environmental Control Centers

Chicago Comprehensive Environmental Control Center

Provides diagnosis and treatment of chronically ill patients (asthma, colitis, arthritis, "brain-fag," depression and other related problems). Training fellowships for physicians and nurses are available. Address all correspondence to Theron G. Randolph, M.D., 505 N. Lake Shore Drive, Chicago, Illinois, 60611, (312) 838-9480.

The Dallas Environmental Center, Dallas, Texas
   consisting of the Brookhaven Medical Center Environmental Control Unit, William J. Rea, M.D., F.A.C.S.-Clinical Associate Professor of Thoracic & Cardiovascular Surgery, University of Texas Southwestern Medical School; the University of Texas at Dallas, Division of Environmental Sciences and North Texas State University, Department of Behavorial Psychology. This center is dedicated to the study of the environmental aspects of health and disease. Fellowships for M.D., D.O., and Ph.Ds are available for this study. Emphasis is placed on patients with problems of air, water, food, and chemical analysis with challenge and testing under controlled conditions. Study of cardiovascular responses, rheumatoid and muscularskeletal responses, gastrointestinal as well as genitourinary and skin problems is available. Emphasis on patient care both in and out of the hospital is maintained. All communication should be addressed to William J. Rea, M.D., 8345 Walnut Hill Lane, Suite 205, Dallas, Texas, 75231, (214) 368-4132.

The Environmental Care Unit, Denver, Colorado
   Presbyterian Denver Hospital, a division of Presbyterian/Saint Luke's Medical Center, 1719 East 19th Avenue, Denver, Colorado, 80218, (303) 839-6475. Since early 1979, the Department of Medicine has operated a 12-room Environmental Care Unit (ECU). The ECU is a self-contained unit within the traditional hospital setting, with its own staff, equipment, and facilities necessary to maintain a controlled environment. It also receives full staff, laboratory and other kinds of support for its unique program of diagnosis and care. The diagnosis in the ECU draws heavily from the fields of both allergy and industrial medicine. Kendall Gerdes, M.D., is the director.

Southeastern Rheumatology and Allergy Center
   Provides comprehensive allergy testing and treatment for inhalants, foods, and chemicals, utilizing controlled environmental

methods. Address all correspondence to Southeastern Rheumatology and Allergy Center, 722 N. Brown Street, Chadbourn, North Carolina, 28431, (919) 654-4614.

Physicians Employing Comprehensive Environmental Control in Isolated Rooms

Dr. John Argabrite
First National Bank Building
P.O. Box 258
Watertown, South Dakota 57301
(605) 886-3144

Drs. Bullock & Carroll
722 N. Brown Street
Chadbourn, North Carolina
   28431
(919) 654-4614

Dr. Steven Cordas
Hurst General Hospital
837 Brown Trail
Hurst, Texas 76021
(817) 266-1327

Environmental Care
   Unit–Presbyterian Hospital
c/o Learning Resource
   Department
1719 East 19th Avenue
Denver, Colorado 80218
303-839-6475

Dr. Harris Hosen
2649 Proctor Street
Port Arthur, Texas 77640
(713) 985-5585

Dr. Joseph Morgan
Bay Clinic
1750 Thompson Road
Coos Bay, Oregon 97420
(503) 269-0333

Drs. Morris & Kroker
Restricted Ward Access Area
for Environmentally Ill Patients
615 S. 10th Street
La Crosse, Wisconsin 54601
(608) 782-2027

To Find Out More . . .

If you are curious about allergy, clinical ecology, bioecologic disorders of body and mind, and nutrition, or if you want to gain a better understanding of how some of us clinical ecologists have made our discoveries and developed our concepts and methods, which have had and will continue to have a major influence on the practice of the healing arts in modern society, you can find these books and articles in your bookstore or library:

Books

Corwin, Alsoph H., Ph.D. "The Rotating Diet and Taxonomy," *Clinical Ecology,* edited by Lawrence D. Dickey, M.D., Springfield, Ill.: Charles C. Thomas, 1976.

Ellis, John, M.D., and Presley, James. Vitamin B$_6$, *The Doctor's Report*. New York: Harper & Row, 1973.

Forman, Robert, Ph.D. *How to Control Your Allergies*. New York: Larchmont Books, 1979.

Golos, Natalie, and Golos, Frances. *If This Is Tuesday—It Must Be Chicken! Or How To Rotate Your Food For Better Health*. Dallas: Human Ecology Research Foundation of the Southwest, 1981.

Hosen, Harris, M.D. *Clinical Allergy (Based on Provocative Testing)*. Available from Dr. Hosen's office at Proctor St., Port Arthur, Texas.

Kaufman, William, M.D., Ph.D. *The Common Form of Joint Dysfunction: Its Incidence and Treatment*. Brattleboro, Vt.: E. L. Hildreth and Co., 1949.

Mandell, Marshall, M.D., and Scanlon, Lynne Waller. *Dr. Mandell's Five-Day Allergy Relief System*. New York: Thomas Y. Crowell, 1979, and Pocket Books, 1980.

Mandell, Fran Gare, M.S. *Dr. Mandell's Allergy-Free Cookbook*. New York: Pocket Books, 1981.

Nikel, Casimir, and Pfieffer, Guy O., M.D. *Household Environments and Chronic Illness*. Springfield, Ill.: Charles C. Thomas, 1980.

Randolph, Theron G., M.D. *Human Ecology and Susceptibility to the Chemical Environment*. Springfield, Ill.: Charles C. Thomas, 1962.

Randolph, Theron G., M.D., and Moss, Ralph W., Ph.D. *An Alternative Approach To Allergies*. New York: Lippincott & Crowell, 1980.

Randolph, Theron G., M.D. "Ecologically Oriented Rheumatoid Arthritis," *Clinical Ecology,* edited by Lawrence D. Dickey, M.D. Springfield, Ill.: Charles C. Thomas, 1976.

Randolph, Theron G., M.D. "Ecologically Oriented Myalgia and Related Musculoskeletal Painful Syndromes." *Clinical Ecology,* edited by Lawrence D. Dickey, M.D. Springfield, Ill.: Charles C. Thomas, 1976.

Rapp, Doris, M.D. *Allergies and Your Family*. New York: Sterling Publishing Co., 1980.

NOTE: This is an abbreviated reading list. Consult the many valuable references in these books and papers.

Rinkel, H. J., Randolph, T. G., and Zeller, M. *Food Allergy.* Springfield, Ill.: Charles C. Thomas, 1951 (available through New England Foundation for Allergic and Environmental Diseases, 3 Brush St., Norwalk, Ct. 06850).

Travis, Nick, and Holladay, Ruth. *The Body Wrecker.* Amarillo, Tex.: Don Quixote Publishing Co., 1981.

Williams, Roger J., Ph.D. *Nutrition Against Disease; Environmental Prevention.* New York: Pitman, 1971.

Zamm, Alfred V., M.D., with Gannon, Robert. *Why Your House May Endanger Your Health.* New York: Simon & Schuster, 1980

Papers

Carroll, Murray F., M.D. "Rheumatoid and Osteoarthritis Controlled by Ecological Management: A Three and One-Half Year Study." Presented to the 12th Advanced Seminar in Clinical Ecology, Key Biscayne, Florida, November 20, 1978.

Kaufman, William, M.D., Ph.D. "The Overall Picture of Rheumatism and Arthritis." *Annals of Allergy* 10 (1952):308.

Kaufman, William, M.D., Ph.D. "Niacinamide Therapy for Joint Motility." *Connecticut State Medical Journal* 17 (1953):584.

Kaufman, William, M.D., Ph.D. "Food-induced Allergic Musculoskeletal Syndromes." *Annals of Allergy* 11 (1953):179.

Kaufman, William, M.D., Ph.D. "Niacinamide, a Most Neglected Vitamin." 1978 Tom Spies Memorial Lecture, *New Dynamics of Preventive Medicine,* International Academy of Preventive Medicine (1981) vol. 6.

Mandell, Marshall, M.D. and Conte, Anthony, M.D. "The Role of Allergy in Arthritis, Rheumatism and Polysymptomatic Cerebral, Visceral and Somatic Disorders: A Double-blind Study." *Journal of the International Academy of Preventive Medicine* (July 1982).

Randolph, Theron G., M.D. "An Ecologic Orientation in Medicine: Comprehensive Environmental Control in Diagnosis and Therapy." *Annals of Allergy* 23 (1965):7.

Zeller, Michael, M.D. "Rheumatoid Arthritis—Food Allergy as a Factor." *Annals of Allergy* 7 (1949):200–205.

Epilogue

A final word to my readers: I sincerely hope that my book has helped you who have lived with the miseries of arthritis—as victims of this often reversible disease or as the caring friends or loved ones of afflicted individuals.

Whatever gains in health and happiness we have been able to make by working together through these pages are a gift from my colleagues and myself. We have been privileged to observe, to recognize the importance of, and to have the opportunity to develop superior methods of diagnosis and treatment for what now are clearly established bioecologic diseases—including arthritis—that seriously affect the physical and mental health of hundreds of millions of our fellow humans.

You and I are greatly indebted to those open-minded, clear-thinking observers and investigators—the trailblazing, pioneering medical ecologists and nutritionists whose inspired concepts, pains-taking efforts, reproducible clinical results, and logical conclusions have permanently changed the perspective and goals of deeply concerned members of all the healing professions.

At the dawn of this Golden Age of bioecologic medicine, with its enormous potential for the welfare of all humanity, our colleagues in the mainstream of today's drug-oriented, ecologically and nutritionally unaware medical establishment have an inescapable ethical and moral responsibility to serve their patients' needs by using the safest and most effective measures to restore and maintain their patients' health without exhausting their financial resources. It is imperative that all physicians become thoroughly informed regarding the concepts, principles, and practices of bioecologic medicine. If this essential sphere of currently available medical knowledge is not at their immediate disposal in their daily practice, their patients will not be treated at the level of professional competence that they deserve.

Index

Action Against Allergy (AAA), 255

Acupuncture, 56

Addictive food allergy, 70, 72–73, 107, 108, 138, 139, 145

Adrenal glands, 238–39

Airborne (natural) allergens, 136–37, 185, 187–88, 206, 215, 232, 253
  diagnostic techniques for, 75–77, 136–38
  questionnaires on susceptibility to, 188–90
  systemic effects of, 65–66, 75
  See also Allergy; *and specific allergens*

Alan Mandell Center for Bio-Ecologic Diseases, 25, 187, 252–53

Alcoholic Beverages
  addiction to, allergic basis of, 73
  evaluation of reactions to, 124–30
  foods used in preparation of (table), 126–29

Alexander, Dale, 244

Alka-Seltzer Gold, 149, 179

Alkaline Salts, Dr. Randolph's, 149

Allergenic extracts, 74–76, 84–85
  See also Sublingual tests

Allergens, *see* Airborne allergens; Chemical allergens; Food allergens

Allergic arthritis
  chemical allergens and, 187–92, 206–16

diagnostic questionnaire for detection of, 95–106

Personal Diet Survey findings and, 109, 130–31

questionnaires on environmental causes of, 187–206

research on, 25–37, 79–87
  See also Allergy

"Allergic resistance," 77

Allergy
  addictive, 70, 72–73, 107, 108, 138, 139, 145
  alcoholic beverages and, 73, 124–30
  cyclic, 70–72, 139
  definition of, 63–64
  fixed, 70, 71, 73–74, 139, 231, 232
  Personal Diet Survey for detection of, 107–31
  physiological mechanisms of, 65–69, 79–80
  questionnaires for detection of, 96–106
  range of symptoms in, 33–36, 64–66, 69
  See also specific diets

American Academy of Allergy, 86

American College of Allergists, 86

American Rheumatism Association, 86

Anderson, Franklin C., 87

Animal dander, *see* Dander

Animal food families, listed, 157–59, 165

Ankylosing spondylitis (AS), 35, 50
Ankylosis, definition of, 45
Antacids, 149
Antibiotics, 160*n,* 233
Antihistamines
  during fasts, 150
  natural, 238
Antimalarial drugs, 55–56
Arachidonic acid, 245
Argabrite, John, 259
Arthritis
  definition of, 41–42
  self-diagnosis of, 87–88
  types of, reviewed, 41–50
  See also Allergic arthritis; *and other specific types*
Arthritis Foundation, 19–20, 83, 86–87, 181, 237–38
Ascorbic acid, 149
  See also Vitamin C
Asphalts, 195
Aspirin, 26, 31, 32, 37, 54, 146, 238
  in lupus, 49
  in rheumatoid arthritis, 44–46
  side effects of, 54
Asthma, 67–68
Aurothioglucose, 55
Azathioprine, 55, 57

Baker's yeast, 234
Barnes, Broda, 153*n*
Barton-Wright, E. C., 238
Beef, 31, 35
Betaine hydrochloride, 240
Bicarbonate of soda, *see* Sodium bicarbonate
Billman, Alice, 257
Biochemical individuality, 59
Blood-vessel walls, leakage through, 51
Brewer's yeast, 233
Bufferin, 29
Bullock, Thurman, 27–30, 85, 86, 252, 259
Bursal sacs, 41
Bursitis, 41, 49–50
Butazolidan (phenylbutazone), 55

Cane sugar, 25, 27–28
Carpal-tunnel syndrome, 18, 243

Carroll, F. Murray, 27–30, 85, 86, 252, 259
Carrots, 31–32
Cartilage
  in normal development of joint, 41–42
  in osteoarthritis, 42–43
  in rheumatoid arthritis, 44–45
Cell wall permeability, 239
Cereal grains, 219
  close relatives of, 156
  in Rotary Diagnostic Diet, 175–78
Chao, I-Tsu, 86
Chemical allergens, 30–31, 37–39, 58, 60, 66, 74, 84, 85, 136–38, 146–48, 185–216, 232–33
  "fasting" from, 206–10
  interaction with dietary allergens, 232–33, 235–36
  questionnaires on environmental presence of, 199–205
  questionnaires on susceptibility to, 188–98, 204–5
  testing arthritis responses to, 210–16
  See also Allergy; *and specific allergens*
"Chemical susceptibility," concept of, 193*n*
Chicago Comprehensive Environmental Control Center, 258
Chicken, 35
Childers, Norman, 34, 246–47
Chlorambucil, 55
Chlorine, 233, 235*n*
Chloroquine, 55–56
Climate, 59, 60
Clinical Ecology (ed. Dickey), 193*n*
Clinoril (sulindac), 46
Coal products, allergy to, 66, 136, 193–94
Coca, Arthur, 147, 179
Cod-liver oil, 244
Columbus County Hospital, North Carolina, 28
Combustion products, allergy to, 193–95
Conte, Anthony, 79, 84–85, 252
Contractures, 47
Cordas, Steven, 259

Corn, 26–27, 35, 80, 233
Corticosteroids, *see* Steroid drugs
Cortisone, 26, 29
See also Steroid drugs
Corwin, Alsoph H., 91
    food-classification system of, 156
Cosmetics, 190, 195
Cottonseed, 191
Cravings, 72–73, 107, 108, 139, 142, 232, 233
Croft, John C., 247
Crustaceans, 156
Cyclic food allergy, 70–72, 139
Cyclophosphamide, 55
Cytotoxic drugs, *see* Immunosuppressive drugs
Cytotoxic testing, 254

Dallas Environmental Center, 258
Dander, 32, 63, 65, 74–76, 136, 137, 190
Degenerative joint disease, *see* Osteoarthritis
Deliberate single-feeding tests (DFTs), 26, 27, 30–32, 34–36, 72, 76, 85–86, 147–48
    hyperreactivity as basis of, 133–34
    reducing diet derived from, 138–39
    self-administered, 133, 171; *and see* Rotary Diagnostic Diet
Deodorants, 196
Derris root, 191–92
Desensitizing allergy treatments (immunotherapy), 36, 77, 83, 85, 215, 238, 254
Detergents, 196
DFTs, *see* Deliberate single-feeding
Diagnostic techniques, 74–77, 83–86, 136–38, 252–55
    and susceptibility to chemicals, 185–216
    See also Deliberate single-feeding tests; Rotary Diagnostic Diet; *and specific techniques*
Dickey, Lawrence D., 76, 193n
Diet
    during "chemical fasting," 208
    low-fat, 245–46
    weight-reduction, 138–39

See also Food Elimination Diet; Lifetime Arthritis-Relief Diet; Nutritional therapies; Personal Diet Survey; Rotary Diversified Diet; Spring-water fast
Digestion process, 239–41
Dimethylsulfoxide (DMSO) treatment, 56
Discoid lupus erythematosis, 49
Disinfectants, 196
Dr. Mandell's Allergy-Free Cook Book (Fran Gare Mandell), 226
Dr. Mandell's Five-Day Allergy Relief System (Mandell and Scanlon), 64, 72, 185
Dong, Collin H., 245–46
Drug treatment, 53–58, 81, 251–52
    for asthma, 68
    in JRA, 47–48
    in lupus, 49
    in rheumatoid arthritis, 45–46, 55, 57
    See also specific drugs
Dust allergies, 32, 38, 58, 76, 136, 189, 206, 233
Dyes, 195

Ecologic units, *see* Environmental-control units
Eliot, W. A., 238
Ellis, John, 18, 237n, 243–44
Enemas, 144, 149, 179
Environmental allergens, *see* Airborne allergens; Chemical allergens; *and specific allergens*
Environmental Care Unit, Denver, Colo., 258
Environmental-control (ecologic) units, 26, 30, 32, 86, 140, 143, 147–48, 210, 257–59
Enzymes in digestion, 239–41
Epsom salts, 149

Fasting
    "chemical," 206–10
    as folk remedy for arthritis, 59
    See also Spring-water fast

Fat in diet, 245–46
Feathers, 190
Fenoprofen, 46, 54–55
Fibers, synthetic, 190, 207
Fish food families, listed, 157–58, 165
Fixed food allergy, 70, 71, 73–74, 139, 231, 232
Flaxseed, 191
Fleets Phospho Soda, 150
Folk remedies, 58–59
Folkers, Karl, 18
Food allergens, 69–74, 84
    in addictive food allergy, 70, 72–73, 107, 108, 138, 139, 145
    building tolerance to, 221–36
    commonest offenders, 134, 155, 170
    in cyclic allergies, 70–72, 139
    diagnostic techniques for, 74–77, 83–86
    in fixed allergies, 70, 71, 73–74, 139, 231, 232
    hidden (list), 233–34
    interaction of environmental allergens with, 232–33, 235–36
    patient's knowledge of, 92
    See also Allergy; Rotary Diversified Diet; *and specific foods*
Food colorings, 234
Food Elimination Diet, 134–35, 137–39, 154–71, 173–74
    basic instructions for, 154–56, 165–68
    environmental precautions for, 140–41
    food-family lists, 157–63
    foods in different families (lists), 164–65
    menu-planning form for, 169
    recording of, 151–53, 168
    sample diet, 170
Food families, 155–69, 218–21
    lists of, 157–65
Ford, Robert Samuelson, 25–27, 82
Fox, Elaine, 237*n*
Fuel oil, 38, 66

Gamma-linolenic acid, 245
Gardner, Robert W., 164*n*

Gas, allergy to, *see* Natural gas
Gerdes, Kendall, 84, 258
Gold injections, 26, 32, 55
Goosefoot family, 168
Gourd family, 156, 167, 219
Gout, 50
Grains, *see* Cereal grains
Grass family, *see* Cereal grains
Grass pollens, 38
Green lipid mussel extract, 247
Guidelines (Billman), 257

Hair analysis, 255
Hansel, French, 76
Henrotin Hospital, Chicago, 26–27
Herbs, *see* Seasonings
Hereditary factors, 51
Hippocrates, 53, 72, 251
Horrobin, David, 237*n*, 244–45
Hosen, Harris, 29, 33–34, 76, 143, 145–46, 154, 259
Human Ecology Action League (HEAL), 256
Human Ecology Foundation of Canada, 256
Human Ecology Research Foundation, 256
Human Ecology Research Foundation of the Southwest, Inc., 256–57
Hydroxychloroquine, 55–56
Hyperreactive state, 133–34
Hypothyroidism (Barnes), 153*n*

Ibuprofen, 46, 54–55
Immune system and allergic reactions, 67, 69, 75
Immunosuppressive (cytotoxic) drugs, 55, 57, 254
Immunotherapy, *see* Desensitizing allergy treatments
Indocin (indomethacin), 46
Indole, NSAIDs derived from, 46
Indomethacin, 46, 54–55
Infectious Diseases (periodical), 57
Inhalants
    chemical, *see* Chemical allergens
    natural, *see* Airborne allergens
Inhalation tests, nasal, 76

Intradermal injections, 75
Ivory soap, 209

Joint Range Index (JRI), 242–43
Joints
    allergen's impact on, 79–80
    in JRA, 46–47
    in lupus, 49
    nonarthritic pain in, 50–51
    normal development of, 41–42
    in osteoarthritis, 42–43
    in rheumatoid arthritis, 43–45
Juvenile rheumatoid arthritis (JRA), 31–32
    general description of, 46–48

Kaufman, William, 237*n*, 238, 241–43
Kroker, George, 86, 87, 234, 259

Laxatives, 144, 149, 150
Lead, 239
Lee, Carleton F., 31–32, 36, 37
    neutralization technique of, 75, 84
Legume family, 167–68
Lifetime Arthritis-Relief Diet, 174, 217–36
    basic principles of, 231–36
    checklist for, 235–36
    permanent phase of, 221–35
    phase one of, 217–21
    sample menus, 222–24
Linoleic acid, 245
Lupus, *see* Systemic lupus erythematosus
Lymphoid radiation therapy, 56–58

McGovern, Joseph J., Jr., 35–36, 164*n*
Magnesium, 244
Magnesium citrate, 150
Mandell, Fran Gare, 226
Marie-Strumpell spondylitis, *see* Ankylosing spondylitis
May, J. M., 248
Mayo Clinic, 87, 146
Medication, *see* Drug treatment
Mercury, 239
Methotrexate, 55, 57
Mildew, 188, 206, 215, 233

Milk allergies, 29, 31, 32
Milk of Magnesia, 149
Minerals
    in diet, 238–39
    in treatment of arthritis, 244, 245
Mold allergies, 32, 38, 58, 60, 75, 76, 136, 137, 188–89, 206, 215, 233
Monoarticular vs. polyarticular JRA, 46
Morgan, Joseph, 259
Morris, Dr. (La Crosse, Wisc.), 259
Motrin (ibuprofen), 46
Mouthwashes, 144, 166
Mustard family, 156, 219–20
Myochrisine (sodium aurothiomalate), 55

Nalfon (fenoprofen), 46
Naprosyn (naproxen), 46
Nasal inhalation tests, 76
Natural gas, 30–32, 37, 38, 66, 93, 136
Natural inhalants, *see* Airborne allergens
Neu, H. C., 57
Neutralization technique, 75, 84
New England Foundation for Allergic and Environmental Diseases, 257
New England Journal of Medicine, 57
New Zealand green lipid mussel extract, 247
Niacinamide (vitamin B_3), 241–43, 245
Nightshade family, 34, 167, 246–47
Nonsteroidal anti-inflammatory drugs (NSAIDs), 46, 54–55
Nutritional therapies, 40, 77, 83, 237–48

Oil products, allergy to, 193–94
Orange juice, 29
Orgotein, 241
Orris root, 190
Osteoarthritis, 28, 84, 85
    definition of, 42–43
Oxygen during fasts, 149–50

Pancreas, function of, 240
Pantothenic acid, 238–39
Paradichlorobenzene, 191–92
Pauciarticular JRA, 46
Penicillamine, 55
Periostium, 41
Personal Diet Survey, 107–31
  feelings and responses to foods, 107–16
  frequency of ingestion, 109, 117–23
  prime suspect list, 130–31
  reactions to alcoholic beverages, 124–30
Petroleum-related products, 30–31, 37, 66, 136, 137, 190, 207, 210, 211
  diagnostic questionnaires on, 193–95
Pfeiffer, Guy O., 76
Phenyl food components (PFC), 164n
Phenylbutazone, 55
Philpott, William, 240
Pine allergy, 198, 206
Plant food families, listed, 160–65
Plastic, 207–8
Pollens, 37, 38, 58, 65, 75, 76, 136, 137, 188, 215
Pollutants, *see* Chemical allergens
Polyarticular vs. monoarticular JRA, 46
Potato, 34, 167
Prednisone, 47–48, 54, 146
Propionic acid, NSAIDs derived from, 46
Prostaglandins, 244–45
Protein, daily intake of, 138–39
Pulse-rate changes, 178–79
Pulse Test, The (Coca), 147, 179
Pyrethrum, 191–92
Pyridoxine (Vitamin B$_6$), 239, 243–44

RA, *see* Rheumatoid arthritis
Radiation therapy, lymphoid, 56–58
Randolph, Theron G., 20–21, 26, 27, 30–32, 37, 80n, 82, 84, 86, 87, 193n, 251, 252, 256, 258
  alkaline-salts recipe of, 149
RAST testing, 254–55

Rea, William J., 86, 146–48, 252, 256, 258
Reich, Carl, 237n, 244
Relief from Arthritis (Croft), 247
Relief of induced reactions, 149–50, 179
Remissions, "spontaneous," 28, 37, 86–87, 147, 181
  in rheumatoid arthritis, 44, 45
Resins, 195
"Resistance, allergic," 77
Reynaud's disease, 69
Rheum, 44
Rheumatism, definition of, 51
Rheumatoid arthritis (RA), 13, 26–28, 34–36, 55, 84, 85, 87, 252
  general description of, 43–46
  total lymphoid radiation for, 57
  See also Juvenile rheumatoid arthritis
Rheumatoid spondylitis, *see* Ankylosing spondylitis
Rinkel, Herbert, 72, 80n, 86, 133–34, 173
  on types of food allergy, 70, 71, 73
Rinkel deliberate feeding test, *see* Deliberate single-feeding test
Rinkel Rotary Diversified Diet, *see* Rotary Diversified Diet
Rose family, 161n
Rotary Diagnostic Diet, 173–84, 232
  blank menu form, 176
  Cycle I of, 174–79
  Cycles II and III of, 180
  keeping records of, 178–79
  sample diet, 177
  summarizing results of, 179, 183–84
Rotary Diversified Diet (RDD), 58, 83, 87, 135–36, 148, 167
  diagnostic form of, *see* Rotary Diagnostic Diet
  See also Food Elimination Diet; Lifetime Arthritis-Relief Diet
Royal jelly, 238

Saccharin, 247
St. Mary's Hospital, Beaumont, Tex., 29
Salicylates, 45

Seasonal arthritis, 37, 187–88
  See also Cyclic arthritis
Seasonings (herbs and spices), 220–21
  for meats, poultry and seafood (table), 225–26
  for vegetables (table), 227–30
Siegel, Jacob, 35, 36
Skin allergies, 68–69
Skin tests for allergy, 74–76, 254, 255
SLE, *see* Systemic lupus erythematosus
Smoking
  and fasting, 141–42
  See also Tobacco smoke
Soaps, 209
Society for Clinical Ecology, 250, 257
Sodium ascorbate, 149
Sodium aurothiomalate, 55
Sodium bicarbonate, 149
  enemas, 144, 149, 179
Sodium urate, 50
Solanine, 246
Solganal (aurothioglucose), 55
Southeastern Chronic Disease Center, Chadburn, N.C., 27–28, 30, 85
Southeastern Rheumatology and Allergy Center, 258–59
Spices, *see* Seasonings
Spondylitis, *see* Ankylosing spondylitis
Spring-water fast, 26–27, 30, 86, 134, 137–53
  basic instructions for, 143–45
  daily record of, 142, 145, 150–53
  environmental precautions for, 140–41
  physician's advice on, 137–38, 140, 145
  remedies for allergic symptoms during, 149–50
  smoking and, 141–42
  Voors case history, 146–48
Steroid (cortisone-related) drugs, 32, 54, 146
  in JRA, 47–48
  in lupus, 49
  side effects of, 54

Stigler, Del, 250, 257
Still's disease, *see* Juvenile rheumatoid arthritis
Stress, 51
Sublingual tests, 84–85, 253
Sugar, 25, 27–28
Sulindac, 46
Superoxide dysmutase, 241
Surgery, 56
  reconstructive, in JRA, 47
Sweeteners, artificial, 247
Symptom key (abbreviations), 184, 192
Symptom(s)
  in determination of allergic arthritis, 95–106
  induced by diet, relief of, 149–50, 179
  varied, allergens as single cause of, 33–36, 64–66, 69
  arthritis as, 36
Synovia
  definition of, 41
  in JRA, 47
  in rheumatoid arthritis, 44
Systemic lupus erythematosus (SLE), 48–49, 55

"Talking Books" program, 255
Tars, 195
Teeth cleaning, 144, 166
Tests, *see* Diagnostic techniques
Tobacco smoke, 136, 137, 186, 191, 208–9
Tolectin (tolmetin sodium), 46
Tolerance to allergens, 221–36
Tomato, 34, 246
Total lymphoid radiation, 56–58

Viruses, 51
Vitamin A, 239, 244
Vitamin B complex, 239
  B$_3$ (niacinamide), 241–43, 245
  B$_6$ (pyridoxine), 239, 243–45
Vitamin C, 149, 160n, 238–39, 244, 245
Vitamin D, 244
Vitamin E, 239, 244
Voors, Charles, case of, 146–48

Water retention, allergic, 145–46
Weed pollen, 37, 38
  See also Pollens
Weight-reduction diet, 138–39
Wilkinson, Richard S., 26
Williams, Roger J., 59*n*
Withdrawal reactions, 72–73, 138, 139, 145, 171

X-ray treatment, lymphoid, 56–58

Yeast, 31–32, 188–89, 233, 234

Zamm, Alfred V., 95*n*
Zeller, Michael, 20–21, 80*n,* 84
Zinc, 240, 244, 245

DR MANDELL'S 5-DAY ALLERGY RELIEF SYSTEM

Dr Marshall Mandell and Lynne Waller Scanlon

Do you — or anyone you know — suffer from any of the following:

compulsive eating ★ depression ★ compulsive drinking ★ hyperactivity ★ migraine ★ asthma ★ arthritis ★ chronic fatigue ★ schizophrenia ★ hypertension ★ clogged sinus ★ eczema ★ duodenal ulcers ★ multiple sclerosis ★ epilepsy.

All these and many more chronic mental, physical and psycho-somatic illnesses may be the result of undiagnosed allergies. Dr Marshall Mandell's remarkable clinically-tested programme provides allergy relief in only 5 days.